THE ALKALINE DIET
COOKBOOK FOR ONE

100+ Recipes to Lose Weight and Get the Benefits of an Alkaline Diet - Alkaline Smoothies Included for Your Way to Vibrant Health - Massive Energy and Natural Weight Loss! Plant-Based Recipes Are Included!

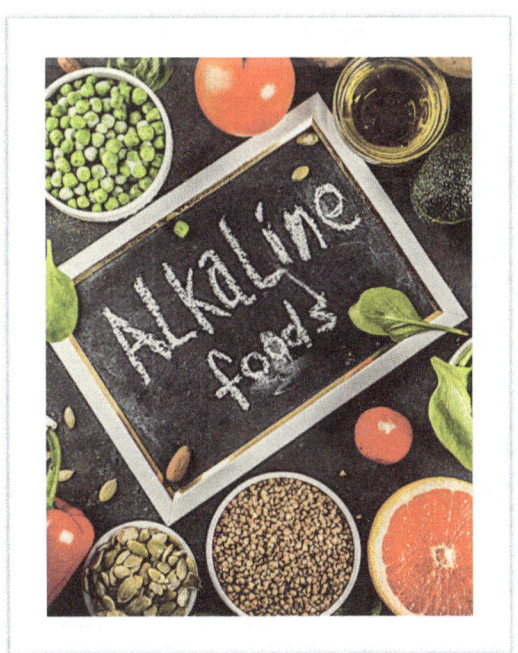

By

Laura Green

TABLE OF CONTENT

INTRODUCTION 6
WHAT SHOULD I KNOW ABOUT THE ALKALINE DIET? 9
BREAKFAST & SMOOTHIES 10
1) Oatmeal and fruit pancakes 11
2) Tofu and mushroom muffins 11
3) Simple white bread 12
4) Quinoa bread 12
5) Courgette and banana bread 12
6) Granola with coconut, nuts and seeds 13
7) Amaranth porridge 13
8) Banana Barley porridge 13
9) Courgette muffins 13
10) Millet Porridge 15
11) Jackfruit Fry vegetable 15
12) Courgette Pancakes 15
13) Squash Hash 15
14) Hemp Seed Porridge 16
15) Veggie Medley 16
16) Pumpkin Spice Quinoa 16
LUNCH 17
17) Baked pumpkin and apples 18
18) Pepperoni and mushroom steak 18
19) Lettuce rolls with avocado and sprouts 19
20) Stir-fried aubergines and peppers 19
21) Nori vegetable rolls 19
22) Tahini beetroot pizza 20
23) Sweet potato slices with artichokes 20
24) Sweet potato stuffed with broccoli and basil pesto 21
25) Cucumber and lentil paste 21
26) Lentil pasta with cashews and artichokes with basil 21
27) Mushrooms stuffed with peppers 22
28) Spaghetti with courgette pesto 22
29) Broccoli and wild rice bowl 23
30) Lentil burgers 23
31) Pumpkin pasta with spaghetti sauce 24
32) Peppers stuffed with vegetables and quinoa 24
33) Aubergine curry with quinoa 24
34) Chili with barbecue bean sauce 25
35) Cooking broccoli and carrots 25
36) Ratatouille 25
37) Fruit and vegetable roast Ritzy 26
38) Brussels sprouts with coconut 26
39) Pasta with basil spinach pesto 26
40) Mushroom and onion risotto 27
41) Vegetable bowl with basil and quinoa 27
42) Spelt sultana biscuits 27

43)	Quinoa and chickpea burgers	28
44)	Chickpea burgers with teff	28
45)	Kamut nut porridge	28
46)	Blueberry, banana and amaranth pancakes	29
47)	Chickpea meatloaf with mushrooms and pepper	29
48)	Fried rice with mushrooms and courgettes	29
49)	Kamut and date porridge	30
50)	Blackberry-flavoured banana and quinoa bars	30
51)	Amaranth and courgette meatballs	30
52)	Spiced chickpeas and cherry tomatoes	31
53)	Herb rice bowl	31
54)	Polenta with amaranth milk and walnuts	31
55)	Breaded peppers with walnuts	31
56)	Pumpkin and amaranth bowl	32
57)	Chickpea and veg hot dogs	32

DINNER..33

58)	Sesame and quinoa pilaf	34
59)	Smoked salmon with fruit sauce	34
60)	Rocket salad with shrimps	35
61)	Easy pizza	35
62)	Spelt bread	36
63)	Green Goddess Bowl with Avocado Dressing	36
64)	Asian sesame dressing and noodles	36
65)	Instant alkaline sushi roll-up	37
66)	Spaghetti filled with quinoa	37
67)	Spelt pasta with spicy aubergine sauce	37
68)	Sesame cabbage with chickpeas	38
69)	Alkaline vegan meatloaf	38
70)	Alkaline pizza crust	39
71)	Alkaline vegan electric chops	39
72)	Walnut meat	40
73)	Electric alkaline steak with mushrooms and cheese	40
74)	Alkaline chickpea tofu	40
75)	Foo Yung Alkaline Electric Egg	41
76)	Alkaline pasta salad	41
77)	Mushrooms 'Chicken shrimps	41
78)	Pizza Margarita	42
79)	Vegetarian electric alkaline lasagne	43
80)	Stuffed aubergines	44
81)	Quinoa pasta with tomato sauce and artichokes	44
82)	Sautéed mushrooms	45
83)	Electric alkaline flat bread	45
84)	Alkaline dinner plate	45
85)	Bowl of alkaline Tahini noodles	46
86)	Balancing alkaline salad	46

SNACKs..47

87)	Spicy Toasted nuts	48
88)	Wheat Crackers	48
89)	Chips potato	48

90)	Courgette Pepper Chips	48
91)	Flat bread	49
92)	Cracker Healthy	49
93)	Tortillas	49
94)	Tortilla chips	51
95)	Onion Rings	51

DESSERTS 52

96)	Green apple smoothie	53
97)	Avocado smoothie	53
98)	Green smoothie	53
99)	Oatmeal and orange smoothie	54
100)	Spicy banana smoothie	54
101)	Blueberry smoothie	54
102)	Raspberry and tofu smoothie	54
103)	Papaya smoothie	55
104)	Peach smoothie	55
105)	Strawberry and beetroot smoothie	55
106)	Grape and chard smoothie	55

AUTHOR BIBLIOGRAPHY 56

CONCLUSIONS 58

© **Copyright 2021 - All rights reserved.**

The content contained within this book may not be reproduced, duplicated or transmitted without direct written permission from the author or the publisher.

Under no circumstances will any blame or legal responsibility be held against the publisher, or author, for any damages, reparation, or monetary loss due to the information contained within this book. Either directly or indirectly.

Legal Notice:

This book is copyright protected. This book is only for personal use. You cannot amend, distribute, sell, use, quote or paraphrase any part, or the content within this book, without the consent of the author or publisher.

Disclaimer Notice:

Please note the information contained within this document is for educational and entertainment purposes only. All effort has been executed to present accurate, up to date, and reliable, complete information. No warranties of any kind are declared or implied. Readers acknowledge that the author is not engaging in the rendering of legal, financial, medical or professional advice. The content within this book has been derived from various sources. Please consult a licensed professional before attempting any techniques outlined in this book.

By reading this document, the reader agrees that under no circumstances is the author responsible for any losses, direct or indirect, which are incurred as a result of the use of information contained within this document, including, but not limited to, — errors, omissions, or inaccuracies.

INTRODUCTION

IMPROVED HEALTH CONDITIONS BY EATING A MORE ALKALINE DIET
An alkaline diet is more effective in treating the following health problems:
- Arthritis
- Diabetes
- Cancer
- Insomnia
- Muscle pain
- Gout
- Bloating

Alkaline water?
Usually, water has a pH of 7, which is referred to as neutral. Alkaline water has a higher pH level, usually 8 to 9. This water helps maintain the alkalinity of the intestines. It is used to cure and treat detoxification, create anti-aging effects, and treat cancer and obesity.

Frequently asked questions about the alkaline diet

Q. How is alkaline food-related to acid reflux?
Acid reflux is when a person feels burning due to the excessive release of HCl in the stomach. Alkaline food is specifically used to treat acid reflux, as it prevents the consumption of all acid-forming foods.

Q. How can alkaline food treat obesity?
By cutting out sugars, complex carbohydrates, saturated fats, the alkaline diet lays out a roadmap for reducing weight and treating obesity.

Q. Does cooking make food alkaline acidic?
No, this is not true at all. We cannot make alkaline food acidic by cooking it. However, adding an acidic ingredient to a meal can make it acidic overall.

Alkaline and acidic foods
Foods that can lower the pH of the intestinal system are called acid-forming foods, while foods that raise the internal pH value are called alkaline-forming foods.

Acid-forming foods
Below is the complete list of acid-forming foods:

- Rice: white, brown, or basmati
- All meat: beef, pork, lamb, fish, and chicken
- Popcorn
- Cornmeal, rye
- Cole
- Cheese
- Pasta
- Wheat Germ
- Alcoholic Beverages
- Coffee and other caffeinated beverages
- Soy sauce

- Sweetened yogurt
- Mustard
- Ketchup
- Refined table salt
- Mayonnaise
- White vinegar
- Nutmeg
- Tobacco

Alkalizing foods
Here is the detailed list of alkalizing foods:
- Beans such as string, soy, lima, green, and snap
- Peas
- Potatoes
- Arrowroot flour
- Cereals such as flax, millet, quinoa, and amaranth
- Nuts such as almonds, fresh coconut, and chestnuts
- Sprouted alfalfa, radish, and chia seeds
- Unsprouted sesame
- Fresh unsalted butter
- Whey
- Plain yogurt
- Fruit juices
- All vegetable juices
- Most herbal teas
- Garlic
- Cayenne pepper
- Jelly
- Most herbs
- Miso
- Most vegetables and unprocessed sea salt
- Most spices
- Vanilla extract
- Sweeteners such as raw, unpasteurized honey, dried sugar cane juice (Sucanat), brown rice syrup
- Brewer's yeast

Chapter 3. What can and cannot be affected by what you eat

Understanding the difference between blood pH, saliva pH, and urine pH

Blood pH:
Blood pH is the acidity of the blood. Its average value is between 7.35 and 7.45.

Urine pH
The expected value of urine pH is between 6 and 7.5. Values below this are dangerous to health.

Saliva pH:
Saliva has a normal pH of 5.6 to 7.9. Therefore, saliva must be slightly neutral or alkaline to function effectively in indigestion.

Testing the pH of urine and saliva
The pH of saliva and urine can be tested at home using acid test strips. For saliva testing, be sure not to eat anything 2 hours before the test. Take some saliva with a cotton swab and place it on the strip. Match the colors with the scale to identify the pH value. Use the same method with urine and dip the strip into the sample to get the color. Consult a health expert if the values are not close to normal.

The 80/20 rule
A diet to be called alkaline should consist of 80 percent alkaline food and 20 percent acidic food. The 80/20 rule is famous because it draws a guideline for setting the bar for alkaline food. Instead of complete abstention, it provides for some relaxation in the 20 percent window.

Acid-forming foods to avoid
- All types of meat, including seafood
- Rice of all kinds
- Bread and crackers purchased at the market.
- Pasta
- Beans
- Artificial sweeteners
- Acidic vegetables such as lemons or limes
- Oatmeal, oats, cornmeal, etc.
- Dairy products

Fermented foods and their role
Fermentation is the process of breaking down food, and it increases the biological value of food. Such foods are great for strengthening the microbiome of the gut. These mainly include miso, tempeh, sauerkraut, kefir, etc. The benefits of fermented foods constitute better digestion, better gut health, and more extended or more accessible storage.

WHAT SHOULD I KNOW ABOUT THE ALKALINE DIET?

HARMFUL EFFECTS OF AN UNBALANCED PH

Maintain a balanced pH is very important. This section will tell you about the fatal consequences of pH changes. If the pH level in your body becomes too alkaline, you will experience a symptom called alkalosis. When the body is put in this condition, you will begin to experience electrolyte loss, liver disease, lower oxygen levels, etc.

Here are some symptoms of alkalosis:
- Tingling in the face
- Breathing problems
- Convulsions
- Sudden onset of muscle spasms
- Spasms
- Light-headedness
- Confusion

On the other hand, if your body becomes too acidic, your body will enter a state of acidosis. There are some risks to acidosis, such as.
- Lethargy
- Shortness of breath
- Fatigue
- Confusion
- Kidney damage
- Insulin resistance
- Diabetes
- Increased risk of heart disease
- Kidney complications
- Lactic imbalance
- Respiratory problems
- Metabolic problems

Acidosis can be caused by a not balanced diet and contains many animal products with few vegetables and fruits.

Here are some symptoms of acidosis:
- Vomiting
- Nausea
- Increased heart rate
- Arrhythmia
- Diarrhea
- Muscle weakness
- Convulsions
- Coughing
- Shortness of breath
- Confusion
- Drowsiness
- Headaches
- Loss of consciousness
- coma

BREAKFAST & SMOOTHIES

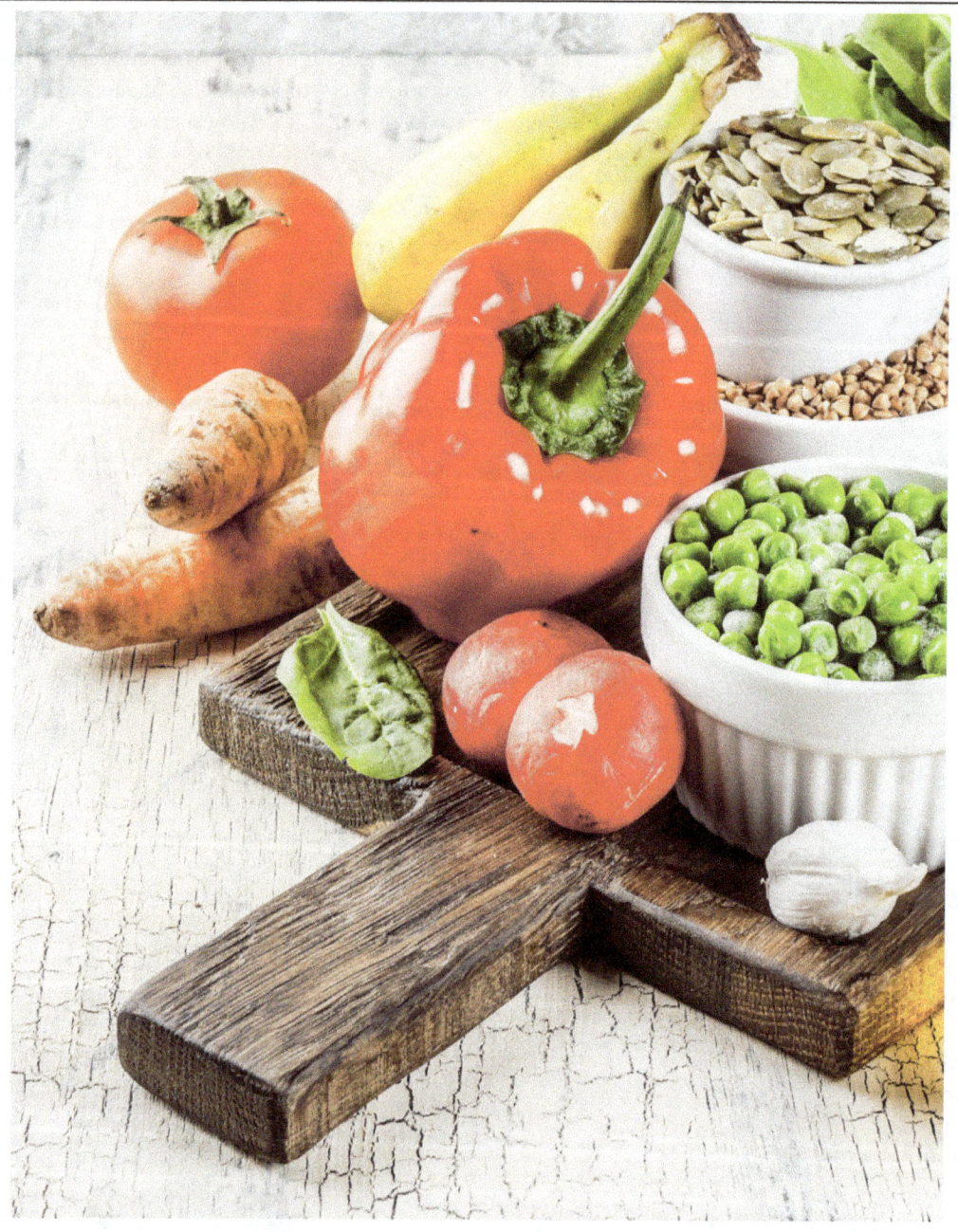

1) Oatmeal and fruit pancakes

Preparation time: 10 minutes **Cooking time**: 15 minutes **Portions**: 3

Ingredients:
- 1 cup rolled oats
- 1 medium banana, peeled and mashed
- ¼-½ cup unsweetened almond milk
- 1 tablespoon organic baking powder

Directions:
- Place all the ingredients except the blackberries in a large bowl and mix until well combined.
- Gently add the blackberries.
- Set the mixture aside for about 5-10 minutes.
- Preheat a large non-stick frying pan over medium-low heat.
- Add about ¼ cup of the mixture and with a spatula, spread into an even layer.

Ingredients:
- 1 tablespoon organic apple cider vinegar
- 1 tablespoon agave nectar
- ½ teaspoon organic vanilla extract
- ½ cup of fresh blackberries
- Immediately, cover the pan and cook for about 2-3 minutes or until golden brown.
- Flip the pancake over and bake for a further 1-2 minutes or until golden brown.
- Repeat with the remaining mixture.
- Serve hot.

2) Tofu and mushroom muffins

Preparation time: 15 minutes **Cooking time**: 30 minutes **Portions**: 6

Ingredients:
- 1 teaspoon of olive oil
- 1½ cups fresh button mushrooms, chopped
- 1 shallot, chopped
- 1 teaspoon chopped garlic
- 1 teaspoon fresh rosemary, chopped
- Freshly ground black pepper, to taste

Directions:
- Preheat the oven to 375 degrees F. Grease a 12-cup muffin tin.
- In a non-stick pan, heat the oil over medium heat and fry the shallots and garlic for about 1 minute.
- Add the mushrooms and cook for about 5-7 minutes, stirring frequently.
- Add the rosemary and black pepper and remove from the heat.
- Set aside to cool slightly.
- In a food processor, add the tofu and the remaining ingredients and pulse until smooth.

Ingredients:
- 1 (12.3ounce) packet of firm silken tofu, drained, pressed and sliced
- ¼ cup unsweetened almond milk
- 2 tablespoons nutritional yeast
- 1 tablespoon arrowroot starch
- ¼ teaspoon ground turmeric
- 1 teaspoon coconut oil, softened
- Transfer the tofu mixture to a large bowl.
- Add the mushroom mixture.
- Divide the tofu mixture evenly between the prepared muffin cases.
- Bake for 20-22 minutes or until a toothpick inserted into the centre comes out clean.
- Remove the muffin tin from the oven and place it on a rack to cool for about 10 minutes.
- Carefully turn the muffins upside down on the wire rack and serve hot.

3) Simple white bread

Preparation time: 10 minutes **Cooking time:** 1 hour and 10 minutes **Portions: 8**

Ingredients:
- 4 cups of spelt flour
- 4 tablespoons of sesame seeds
- 1 teaspoon of bicarbonate of soda

Ingredients:
- ¼ teaspoon of sea salt
- 10-12 drops of liquid stevia
- 2 cups plus 2 tablespoons of unsweetened almond milk

Directions:
- Preheat oven to 350 degrees F. Line a 9x5-inch baking dish with greased baking paper.
- In a large bowl, add all the ingredients and, using a fork, mix until well combined.
- Transfer the mixture evenly into the prepared baking tin.
- Bake for about 70 minutes or until a toothpick inserted into the centre comes out clean.
- Remove from the oven and place the tray on a wire rack to cool for at least 10 minutes.
- Carefully invert the loaf onto the rack to allow it to cool completely before slicing.
- Using a sharp knife, cut the loaf into slices of the desired size and serve.

4) Quinoa bread

Preparation time: 10 minutes **Cooking time:** 1 ½ hours **Portions: 12**

Ingredients:
- ¼ cup chia seeds
- 1 cup of alkaline water, divided by
- 1¾ cup uncooked quinoa, soaked overnight and rinsed
- ½ teaspoon of bicarbonate of soda

Ingredients:
- ¼ teaspoon of sea salt
- ¼ cup of olive oil
- 1 tablespoon fresh lemon juice

Directions:
- In a bowl, soak the chia seeds in ½ cup of water overnight.
- Preheat the oven to 320 degrees F. Line a baking tray with baking paper.
- In a food processor, add the chia seed mixture and the remaining ingredients and pulse for about 3 minutes.
- Place the bread mixture evenly in the prepared baking tin.
- Bake for about 1½ hours or until a toothpick inserted into the centre comes out clean.
- Remove the tray from the oven and place it on a rack to cool for about 10 minutes.
- Carefully invert the loaf onto the rack to allow it to cool completely before slicing.
- Using a sharp knife, cut the loaf into slices of the desired size and serve.

5) Courgette and banana bread

Preparation time: 15 minutes **Cooking time:** 45 minutes **Portions: 6**

Ingredients:
- ½ cup almond flour, sifted
- 1½ teaspoons of bicarbonate of soda
- ½ teaspoon cinnamon powder
- ¼ teaspoon ground cardamom

Ingredients:
- 1/8 teaspoon clove powder
- 1½ cups banana, peeled and sliced
- ¼ cup almond butter, softened
- 2 teaspoons of organic vanilla extract
- 1 cup of courgettes, chopped and squeezed

Directions:
- Preheat oven to 350 degrees F. Grease a 6x3-inch baking dish.
- In a large bowl, add the flour, baking soda and spices and with a fork, mix well.
- In another bowl, add the banana and use a fork to mash it completely.
- In the bowl of the banana, add the almond butter and vanilla extract and beat until well combined.
- Add the flour mixture and stir until just combined.
- Gently add the grated courgettes.
- Pour the flour mixture evenly into the prepared baking tin.
- Bake for about 40-45 minutes or until a toothpick inserted into the centre comes out clean.
- Remove from the oven and place the tray on a wire rack to cool for at least 10 minutes.
- Carefully turn the bread upside down on the rack to cool completely before slicing.

6) Granola with coconut, nuts and seeds

Preparation time: 15 minutes **Cooking time**: 23 minutes **Portions**: 8

Ingredients:
- ½ cup unsweetened coconut flakes
- 1 cup raw almonds
- 1 cup of raw walnuts
- ½ cup of raw, shelled sunflower seeds
- ¼ cup of coconut oil

Ingredients:
- ½ cup maple syrup
- 1 teaspoon organic vanilla extract
- ½ cup sultanas
- ½ cup black sultanas
- Sea salt, to taste

Directions:
- Preheat the oven to 275 F. Line a large baking tray with baking paper.
- In a food processor, add the coconut flakes, almonds, nuts and seeds and pulse until finely chopped.
- Meanwhile, in a medium non-stick frying pan, add the oil, maple syrup and vanilla extract and cook for 3 minutes over medium-high heat, stirring constantly.
- Remove from the heat and immediately stir in the nut mixture.
- Transfer the mixture onto the prepared baking tray and distribute it evenly.
- Cook for about 25 minutes, stirring twice.
- Remove the pan from the oven and immediately stir in the sultanas.
- Sprinkle with a little salt.
- With the back of a spatula, flatten the surface of the mixture.
- Set aside to cool completely.
- Then, break the granola into uniformly sized pieces.
- Serve this granola with your choice of non-dairy milk and fruit toppings.
- To store, transfer this granola to an airtight container and keep in the fridge.

7) Amaranth porridge

Preparation time: 5 minutes. **Cooking time**: 30 minutes. **Portions**: 2

Ingredients:
- 2 cups coconut milk
- 2 cups alkaline water
- 1 cup of administrator

Ingredients:
- 2 tbsps. Coconut oil
- 1 tbsp. land cinnamon

Directions:
- In a bowl, mix the milk with the water and then boil the milk.
- You put in the amaranth and then reduce the heat and make milk.

8) Banana Barley porridge

Preparation time: 15 minutes. **Cooking time**: 5 minutes. **Portions**: 2

Ingredients:
- 1 glass divided unsweetened coconut milk
- 1 small bernard cut into slices
- 1/2 cup barley

Ingredients:
- 3 drops liquid stevia.
- 1/4 cup chopped coconuts

Directions:
- In a bowl, properly mix barley with half the coconut milk and stevia.
- Cover the bowl and leave to rest for about 6 hours.
- In a saucepan, mix the barley mixture with the coconut milk.
- Coook for about 5 minutes on moderate hat.
- Then top with chopped walnuts and bernard.
- Serve.

9) Courgette muffins

Preparation time: 10 minutes. **Cooking time**: 25 minutes. **Portions**: 16

Ingredients:
- 1 tbsp. ground flaxseed
- 3 tbsps. Alkaline water
- 1/4 inch walnut
- 3 medium over-ripe banas
- 2 small grated zucchinis

Ingredients:
- 1/2 cup coco walnut milk
- 1 tsp. extract of vanilla
- 2 cups coconut flour
- 1 tbsp. baking powder
- 1 teaspoon of cinnamon 1/4 teaspoon of sea salt

Directions:
- Set the temperature of your oven to 375°F.
- Grill the muffler tray with the appropriate cover.
- In a bowl, mix the flaxsed with the water.
- In a glass tumbler, massh the bananas and remaining ingredients.
- Mix thoroughly and then divide the mixture into muffin moulds.
- Bake for 25 minutes.
- Serve.

10) Millet Porridge

Preparation time: 10 minutes. **Cooking time:** 20 minutes. **Portions: 2**

Ingredients:
- ✓ Sea salt
- ✓ 1 tbsp. finely chopped coconuts.
- ✓ 1/2 cup unsweetened coconut milk

Directions:
- ❖ Saute the millet in a non-stick skillet for about 3 minutes.
- ❖ Add salt and water, then stir.
- ❖ Allow the meal to rest and reduce the amount of salt.

Ingredients:
- ✓ 1/2 cup of millet rinsed and millet draned
- ✓ 1-1/2 cups water alkaline
- ✓ 3 Drops liquid stevia
- ❖ Cook for about 15 minutes, then add the other ingredients. Stylize.
- ❖ Cook the apple for a further 4 minutes.
- ❖ Serve the meal with a garnish of hazelnuts chopped.

11) Jackfruit Fry vegetable

Preparation time: 5 minutes. **Cooking time:** 5 minutes. **Portions: 6**

Ingredients:
- ✓ 2 onions small finely chopped
- ✓ 2 cups tomatoes chopped cherry finely
- ✓ 1/8 tablespoon cassava butter
- ✓ 1 tablespoon olive oil

Directions:
- ❖ In a fat pan, fry onions and bell peppers for about 5 minutes.
- ❖ Add the tomatoes and mix.
- ❖ Coook for 2 minutes.

Ingredients:
- ✓ 2 seeded and chopped red bell peppers
- ✓ 3 cups firm jackfruit with seeds and chopped
- ✓ 1/8 teaspoon cayenne pepper
- ✓ 2 tbsps. Chopped fresh basil leaves Salt
- ❖ Then add the juice, pepper, salt and turmeric.
- ❖ Cook for about 8 minutes.
- ❖ Garnish the meal with basil leaves.
- ❖ Serve hot.

12) Courgette Pancakes

Preparation time: 15 minutes. **Cooking time:** 8 minutes. **Portions: 8**

Ingredients:
- ✓ 12 tablespoons of alkaline water
- ✓ 6 great zucchini grateds
- ✓ Sea salt
- ✓ 4 tbsp. chopped Flax Seeds

Directions:
- ❖ In a bowl, mix together the water and flax and set aside.
- ❖ Put our food in a large non-stick container and then place it in a cooking container.
- ❖ Add the glass of milk, the glass of wine and the glass of pumpkin.
- ❖ Coook for 3 minutes then transfer the courgettes into a large boge.

Ingredients:
- ✓ 2 tsps. Olive oil
- ✓ 2 finely chopped jalapeño peppers
- ✓ 1/2 cup finely chopped scallions

- ❖ Add the flax and shallot mixture and then mix everything together.
- ❖ Preheat a grill and then grease it well with oil.
- ❖ Pour 1/4 zuchini mixture into a griddle and bake for 3 minutes.
- ❖ Turn side carefully then coook for 2 more minutes.
- ❖ Repeat the procedure with the rest of the mass in random order.
- ❖ Serve.

13) Squash Hash

Preparation time: 2 mnutes. **Cooking time:** 10 minutes. **Portions: 2**

Ingredients:
- ✓ 1 tsp. onion powder.
- ✓ 1/2 cup finely chopped onion

Directions:
- ❖ By using paper towels, you can get an extra moisture from the spaghetti squash.
- ❖ Put the pumpkin in a bowl, then add the salt, onion and onion powder.
- ❖ Stir well to mix everything.
- ❖ Spray a non-stick cooking skillet with coooking spray that place il over moderate heat.

Ingredients:
- ✓ 2 cups of spaghetti squash
- ✓ 1/2 tsp sea salt
- ❖ Add the spaghetti squash.
- ❖ Coook the squash for 5 minutes.
- ❖ Crush the chestnuts with a spatula.
- ❖ Coook formatis of 5 minutes until the desired crispness is reached.
- ❖ Serve.

14) Hemp Seed Porridge

Preparation time: 5 minutes.   **Cooking time**: 5 minutes.   **Portions**: 6

Ingredients:
- 3 cups cooked hemp sed
- 1 packet Stevia

Ingredients:
- 1 cup coco of walnut milk

Directions:
- In a bowl, mix the milk and nut milk for about 5 minutes.
- Remove the pan from the heat and add the stevia. Stylize.
- Serve in 6 bowls.
- Enjoy.

15) Veggie Medley

Preparation time: 5 mnutes.   **Cooking time**: 10 minutes.   **Portions**: 2

Ingredients:
- 1 seed and 1 bacon
- 1/2 cup lime juice
- 2 tablespoons of fresh cilantro
- 1/2 tsp. cumin
- 1 teaspoon sea salt
- 1 wooden jacket

Ingredients:
- 1/2 cup of courgettes
- 1 cup halved cherry tomatoes
- 1/2 cup sliced mushrooms
- 1 cup coooked broccoli florets
- 1 sweet onion chopped

Directions:
- Spray a little paint with stick pan with cooking spray and then put it all over the body.
- Add the butter, tomatoes, chilli, grapes, pumpkin, peanut butter and mushroms.
- Cook for about 7 minutes as you stir from time to time.
- Add the cumin and caraway and then the pepper.
- Cook for a further 3 minutes, stirring.
- Take the pan off the heat and add the lime juice.
- Serve.

16) Pumpkin Spice Quinoa

Preparation time: 10 minutes.   **Cooking time**: 0 minutes.   **Portions**: 2

Ingredients:
- 1 cup of cooked quinoa
- 1 cup unsweetened coconut milk
- 1 large mashed banana

Ingredients:
- 1/4 cup pumpkin pureee
- 1 tsp. pumpkin spice
- 2 teaspoons of chia seds

Directions:
- In a container, mix all the ingredients.
- Close the lid and then close the container to mix.
- Refrigerate overnight.
- Serve.

LUNCH

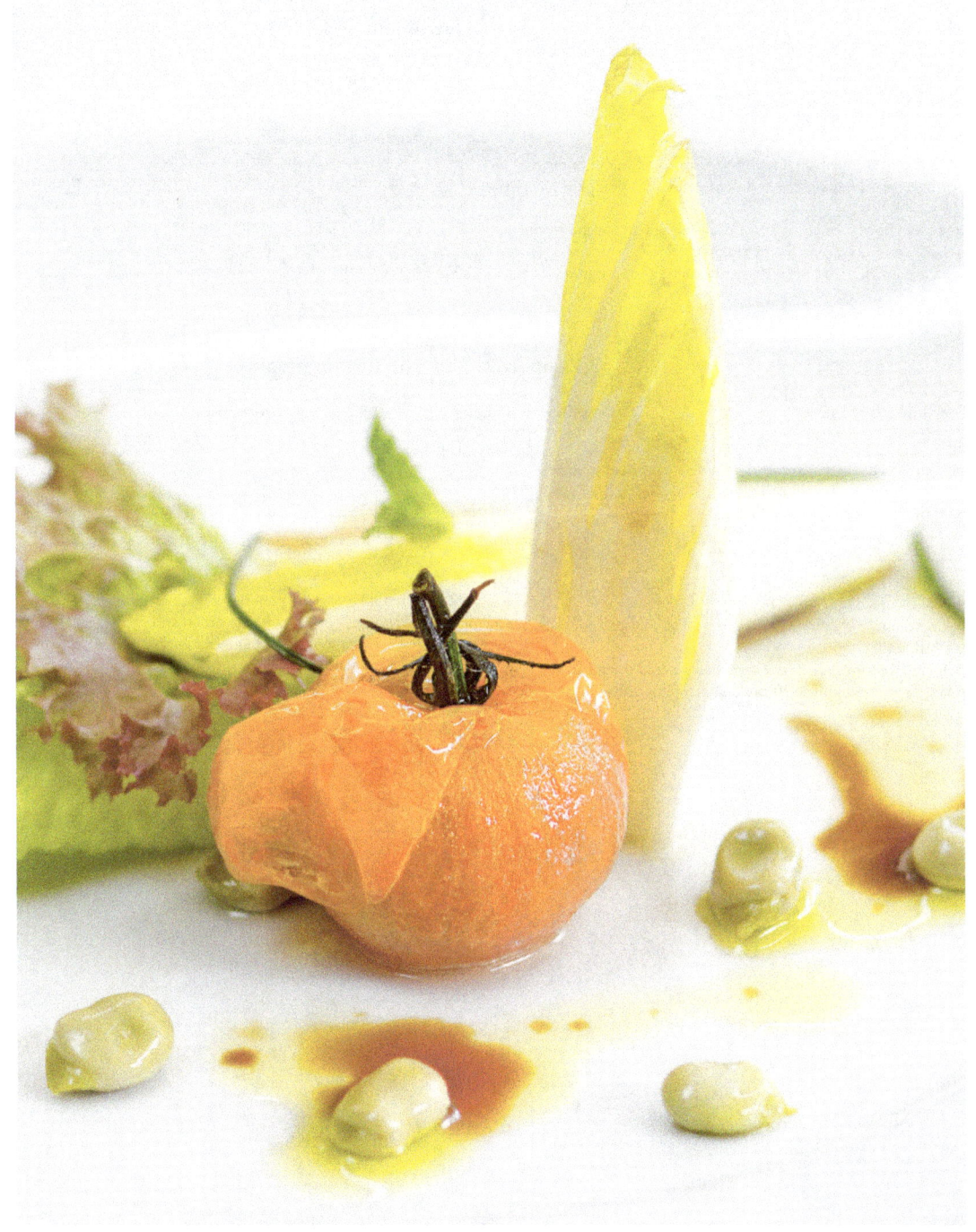

17) Baked pumpkin and apples

Preparation time: 10 minutes **Cooking time**: 35 minutes **Portions**: 2

Ingredients:
- 1½ pounds (680 g) butternut squash, peeled, seeded and cut into pieces
- 2 apples, core, cut into ½ inch pieces
- 2 tablespoons agave syrup

Directions:
- Turn on the oven, then set it to 375°F (190°C) and let it preheat.
- Meanwhile, take a baking tray and then spread the pumpkin pieces on it.
- Take a small bowl, pour in the oil, stir in the salt and allspice until combined, then pour over the pumpkin pieces.
- Cover the pan with aluminium foil and bake for 20 minutes.

Ingredients:
- ½ teaspoon of sea salt
- 2 tablespoons of grape oil

- Meanwhile, place the apple pieces in a medium bowl, drizzle with the agave syrup and stir until coated.
- When the pumpkin is cooked, discard the pan, pour the spoonful into the bowl containing the apple and then stir until combined.
- Spread the apple and pumpkin mixture evenly over the baking tray and then continue baking for 15 minutes.
- Serve immediately.

18) Pepperoni and mushroom steak

Preparation time: 10 minutes **Cooking time**: 10 minutes **Portions**: 2

Ingredients:
- 2 caps of portabella mushrooms, cut into thick slices ⅛ inch
- ½ cup of sliced green peppers
- ½ cup of sliced white onions
- ½ cup of sliced red peppers
- ¼ cup of alkaline sauce
- ½ teaspoon of sea salt

Directions:
- Take a medium bowl, put the sauce in, add all the seasonings and then whisk until combined.
- Add the mushroom slices, sauté until coated, and then leave to marinate for a minimum of 30 minutes, sautéing halfway through.

Ingredients:
- ½ tablespoon of onion powder
- ½ teaspoon dried oregano
- ½ teaspoon dried thyme
- ½ tablespoon of grape oil
- 2 spelt focaccias, toasted

- Then take a frying pan, put it over medium-high heat, add the oil and when it is hot, add the onion and pepper and cook for 3 to 5 minutes until they are tender-crispy.
- Add the mushroom slices, stir until combined and continue cooking for 5 minutes.
- Distribute the vegetables evenly between the sandwiches, roll them up and serve.

19) Lettuce rolls with avocado and sprouts

Preparation time: 10 minutes **Cooking time:** 0 minutes **Portions: 2**

Ingredients:
- ½ cup cherry tomatoes, halved
- 1 avocado, peeled, stoned, sliced
- ½ cup of sprouts
- ½ medium white onion, peeled, sliced
- 2 large lettuce leaves

Directions:
- Take a small bowl, add the lime juice, add salt and pepper and then mix until combined.
- Take a medium bowl, place all the vegetables except the lettuce, drizzle with the lime juice mixture and then toss until mixed.

Ingredients:
- 2 tablespoons of lime juice
- ½ tablespoon of sultanas
- ¼ teaspoon of salt
- ⅛ teaspoon of cayenne pepper

- Place a lettuce leaf on a plate, cover it with half of the vegetable mixture and then roll it up tightly.
- Repeat with the other lettuce wrap and then serve.

20) Stir-fried aubergines and peppers

Preparation time: 10 minutes **Cooking time:** 5 minutes **Portions: 2-4**

Ingredients:
- 3 tablespoons avocado oil
- 3 cups diced aubergine (about three quarters of an aubergine)
- 2 tablespoons of coconut amino acids
- 2 cloves of garlic, crushed
- ½ teaspoon of sea salt

Directions:
- Add the aubergines, coconut amino acid, garlic, salt and pepper and fry for 3-5 minutes, or until the aubergines are soft.

Ingredients:
- ½ teaspoon freshly ground black pepper
- ½ orange pepper, diced
- ½ yellow pepper, diced
- ½ red pepper, diced
- Shallots and/or chopped sesame seeds, for garnish (optional)

- Reduce the heat to low, add the peppers and stir just long enough for everything to be coated.
- Remove from the heat, transfer to 2 large or 4 small plates, and serve garnished with scallions and/or sesame seeds (if using).

21) Nori vegetable rolls

Preparation time: 10 minutes **Cooking time:** 0 minutes **Serves 2 large rolls**

Ingredients:
- 1 avocado, pitted and cut in half
- ¼ cup of fresh coriander leaves
- 2 tablespoons freshly squeezed lemon juice
- ½ to 1 jalapeño
- ¼ teaspoon of sea salt
- 2 leaves of green cabbage

Directions:
- In a blender, blend together the avocado, cilantro, lemon juice, jalapeño and salt until smooth.
- Roll out 1 leaf of green collard and place 1 sheet of nori on top.
- Spread half of the avocado and jalapeño mixture in the centre.

Ingredients:
- 2 sheets of nori
- ½ red pepper, sliced
- ½ orange pepper, sliced
- ½ yellow pepper, sliced
- ½ cup chopped purple cabbage
- 2 tablespoons chopped fresh coriander leaves

- Take half the peppers, cabbage and cilantro and place them in the centre of the nori sheet on top of the avocado and jalapeño cream. Roll up like a burrito. Repeat with the remaining collard leaves, nori, pepper, cabbage and cilantro.
- Enjoy each roll whole or halved.

22) *Tahini beetroot pizza*

Preparation time: 10 minutes **Cooking time**: 15 minutes **Portions: 4 small pieces**

Ingredients:
- For the crust:
- 1¼ cup almond flour
- 3 tablespoons of coconut oil
- ½ teaspoon of sea salt
- ½ teaspoon of garlic powder
- For the spread of beetroot Tahini:
- 2 beets, peeled and diced
- 1 tablespoon tahini

Directions:
- Preheat the oven to 375°F (190°C). Line a baking tray with baking paper.
- Preparing the crust
- In a small bowl, mix together the almond flour, coconut oil, salt and garlic powder until well combined.
- Transfer to the prepared baking tray and press the dough into a ball.

Ingredients:
- 1 tablespoon avocado oil
- 1 tablespoon freshly squeezed lemon juice
- 2 garlic cloves
- ⅛ teaspoon of sea salt
- Pinch of freshly ground black pepper
- For mounting:
- Mushrooms, red onions, dandelions, asparagus, jalapeños, artichokes, rocket, broccoli, basil, dulse flakes (optional condiments)

- Lay another sheet of parchment paper over the ball and use a rolling pin to roll out the dough on the parchment paper into a 7 by 7 inch square.
- Bake for about 14 minutes, until the edges turn golden brown.
- To prepare the Tahini beetroot puree
- Meanwhile, in a food processor, process the beetroot, tahini, avocado oil, lemon juice, garlic, salt and pepper until thickened. Adjust seasonings as necessary.
- To assemble
- When the crust is ready, spread the beetroot tahini evenly over it, top the pizza with your favourite alkaline vegetables, cut into 4 slices and enjoy.

23) *Sweet potato slices with artichokes*

Preparation time: 5 minutes **Cooking time**: 45 minutes **Portions: 8 pieces**

Ingredients:
- 2 unpeeled sweet potatoes, cut into 4 (¼ inch thick) lengthwise
- 1 red pepper, cut into quarters
- 6 teaspoons of avocado oil, divided by
- ½ teaspoon of salt, plus 1 pinch

Directions:
- Preheat the oven to 350°F (180°C). Line a baking tray with baking paper.
- Transfer the sweet potato and pepper to the prepared baking tray and drizzle with 2 teaspoons of avocado oil, the pinch of salt and the pinch of pepper.
- Bake for 30 minutes. Turn them over and put them back in the oven for another 15 minutes.

Ingredients:
- ¼ teaspoon freshly ground black pepper, plus 1 pinch
- 1 (14-ounce / 397-g) may artichoke hearts
- 2 garlic cloves

- In a food processor, puree the roasted red pepper, remaining 4 teaspoons avocado oil, remaining ½ teaspoon salt, remaining ¼ teaspoon black pepper, artichoke hearts and garlic until well combined but still chunky. Adjust seasonings as needed.
- Cover the sweet potato slices with the cream and enjoy.

24) Sweet potato stuffed with broccoli and basil pesto

Preparation time: 10 minutes **Cooking time:** 1 hour 15 minutes **Servings:** 2 potatoes

Ingredients:
- 2 large sweet potatoes
- 2 1/2 cups of broccoli
- 2 ½ cups of almonds
- ½ cup of fresh basil leaves
- ¼ cup onion

Directions:
- Preheat the oven to 350ºF (180ºC).
- Pierce the sweet potatoes all over with a fork. Place the sweet potatoes on a baking tray and bake for 1 hour and 15 minutes, or until soft.
- Meanwhile, prepare the pesto. In a food processor, chop the broccoli, almonds, basil, onion, garlic, avocado oil, nutritional yeast and salt until the broccoli and almonds are chopped into small pieces. Adjust the seasonings as necessary.

Ingredients:
- 2 garlic cloves
- 2 tablespoons of avocado oil
- ¼ cup of nutritional yeast
- ½ teaspoon of sea salt

- When the potatoes are ready, cut them in half lengthwise and gently remove the inside of the potato, taking care not to tear the skin; add the baked potato filling to a medium bowl and add the pesto; mix gently.
- Divide the mixture in half, add each half to the two empty potato skins and serve.

25) Cucumber and lentil paste

Preparation time: 5 minutes **Cooking time:** 0 minutes **Portions:** 1-2

Ingredients:
- ⅓ cup of avocado oil
- 2 tablespoons apple cider vinegar
- 2 tablespoons of water
- ½ teaspoon dried oregano
- ¼ to ½ teaspoon of sea salt
- ¼ teaspoon of ground black pepper
- 2 small fresh basil leaves, chopped

Directions:
- In a small bowl, whisk together the avocado oil, vinegar, water, oregano, salt, pepper and basil until well combined. Adjust the seasonings to your liking.

Ingredients:
- 1 cup cooked lentils
- 1 cup of cooked green lentil paste
- ½ cup of chopped, unpeeled cucumber
- ¼ cup thinly sliced onion
- 5 to 10 small basil leaves, for garnish (optional)

- Add the cooked lentils and pasta to the serving bowl and stir gently to distribute them evenly. Add the cucumbers and onions, drizzle with the dressing and garnish with the basil leaves (if using).
- Transfer to 1 large or 2 small plates and enjoy.

26) Lentil pasta with cashews and artichokes with basil

Preparation time: 5 minutes **Cooking time:** 10 minutes **Portions:** 2-4

Ingredients:
- 2 cups of red lentil paste
- 1¼ cup raw cashews
- ¾ cup of almond milk
- 1 tablespoon freshly squeezed lemon juice
- 3 garlic cloves
- 1 tablespoon nutritional yeast

Directions:
- Cook the pasta according to the package directions.
- Meanwhile, prepare the sauce. In a high-speed blender, blend together the cashews, almond milk, lemon juice, garlic, nutritional yeast, avocado oil, salt and pepper until smooth.

Ingredients:
- 1 tablespoon avocado oil
- ½ teaspoon of sea salt
- ¼ teaspoon freshly ground black pepper
- 1 tin of chopped artichoke hearts
- 1 bunch of fresh basil, cut into long strips (approx. 1 cup)

- Transfer the drained pasta to a large bowl with the sauce, artichokes and basil. Stir gently until well combined, transfer to 2 large or 4 small plates and enjoy.

27) Mushrooms stuffed with peppers

Preparation time: 10 minutes **Cooking time:** 20 minutes **Portions:** 2

Ingredients:
- 2 large portobello mushrooms
- Avocado oil, for rubbing
- Sea salt
- Freshly ground black pepper
- ½ red pepper, diced
- ½ orange pepper, diced
- ½ yellow pepper, diced

Ingredients:
- ¼ cup diced red onion
- 2 cloves of garlic, crushed
- 2 teaspoons of avocado oil
- ½ teaspoon of sea salt
- ½ teaspoon freshly ground black pepper

Directions:
- Preheat the oven to 350°F (180°C). Line a baking tray with baking paper.
- Rinse and dry the mushrooms quickly. Remove the stalks and, with the tip of a spoon, remove the black gills. Rub the mushrooms all over with avocado oil and sprinkle with salt and pepper.
- Transfer the mushrooms to the prepared baking tray and bake for 15-20 minutes, or until the mushrooms are as soft as you like.
- Meanwhile, in a small bowl, mix together the peppers, onion, garlic, avocado oil, salt and pepper until well combined.
- Remove the mushrooms from the oven and discard the accumulated liquid.
- Divide the stuffing mixture evenly between the 2 mushrooms and serve immediately.

28) Spaghetti with courgette pesto

Preparation time: 20 minutes **Cooking time:** 50 minutes **Portions:** 2

Ingredients:
- 1 spaghetti squash
- 2 teaspoons of avocado oil
- Sea salt
- Freshly ground black pepper
- 1 courgette, peeled
- 2 cabbage stalks, chopped
- ½ cup of raw cashews

Ingredients:
- ¼ cup chopped onion
- 2 tablespoons of avocado oil
- 1 tablespoon freshly squeezed lemon juice
- 1 tablespoon nutritional yeast
- 2 garlic cloves
- ½ teaspoon of sea salt

Directions:
- Preheat the oven to 350°F (180°C). Line a baking tray with baking paper.
- Halve the spaghetti lengthwise, remove the seeds, rub the inner and outer edges of both halves with avocado oil, sprinkle with salt and pepper and place on a baking tray. Bake for 45-50 minutes, or until tender.
- Meanwhile, in a food processor, process the courgettes, cabbage, cashews, onion, avocado oil, lemon juice, nutritional yeast, garlic and salt until well combined. Adjust the seasonings as necessary.
- Using a fork, scrape the inside of the pumpkin into long strands. Transfer to a medium bowl.
- Add the pesto and stir gently until well combined. Transfer to 2 plates or bowls and enjoy.

29) Broccoli and wild rice bowl

Preparation time: 10 minutes **Cooking time:** 20 minutes **Portions:** 4

Ingredients:
- 1 cup chopped broccoli florets
- 6 garlic cloves, peeled
- 1 teaspoon avocado oil
- Pinch of sea salt
- Pinch of black pepper
- Pinch of garlic powder
- 6 roasted garlic cloves (from above)
- 1 cup raw cashews
- 1 cup of water
- ½ teaspoon avocado oil

Ingredients:
- ½ teaspoon apple cider vinegar
- ¼ teaspoon of garlic powder
- ¼ to ½ teaspoon of sea salt
- Pinch of freshly ground black pepper
- 1 cup cooked wild rice
- ¼ cup slivered almonds
- 2 tablespoons diced onion
- ½ cup of chopped cabbage tops

Directions:
- Preheat the oven to 400°F (205°C). Line a baking tray with baking paper.
- In a small bowl, mix the broccoli and garlic with the avocado oil to coat. Season with the salt, pepper and garlic powder and transfer to the prepared baking tray.
- Roast the broccoli and garlic for 15-20 minutes, or until the broccoli is soft and slightly crispy.
- In a high-speed blender, blend together the roasted garlic cloves, cashews, water, avocado oil, vinegar, garlic powder, salt and pepper until smooth. Adjust seasonings as needed.
- In a serving bowl, mix the cooked rice with the roasted broccoli, almond slivers, onion and cabbage leaves. Stir in the dressing and enjoy.

30) Lentil burgers

Preparation time: 15 minutes **Cooking time:** 30 minutes **Portions:** 4

Ingredients:
- ½ cup dried lentils (equal to 1 cup cooked)
- ½ cup of almond flour
- ½ teaspoon of sea salt
- ½ teaspoon freshly ground black pepper
- ½ cup diced onion

Ingredients:
- ½ cup chopped coriander leaves
- ½ to 1 jalapeño, diced
- 2 cloves of garlic, crushed
- 1 tablespoon of coconut flour
- 1 tablespoon avocado oil

Directions:
- Prepare the dried lentils according to the packet instructions. Set aside to cool.
- In a medium bowl, mix together the cooled lentils, almond meal, salt, pepper, onion, cilantro, jalapeño and garlic until well combined.
- In a food processor, process half of the lentil mixture to a paste-like consistency.
- Return the processed lentil mixture to the bowl with the other half of the mixture and stir until well combined. The mixture should be very moist, so stir in the coconut flour to help it hold together.
- Take a quarter of the mixture, squeeze it in your hand and flatten it with your palms into a small hamburger. Repeat to make 3 more patties with the remaining lentil mixture.
- In a large skillet over medium-high heat, heat avocado oil. Add burgers; cook 4 to 6 minutes on each side, or until golden brown, turning gently; and serve.

31) Pumpkin pasta with spaghetti sauce

Preparation time: 15 minutes **Cooking time**: 1 hour and 5 minutes **Portions**: 2

Ingredients:
- ✓ 2 cups of spiral spaghetti
- ✓ 2 tablespoons plus 1 teaspoon of coconut oil
- ✓ ¼ onion, chopped
- ✓ 2 teaspoons of sea salt, divided
- ✓ 1 teaspoon chopped garlic

Directions:
- ❖ Preheat the oven to 350°F (180°C).
- ❖ To roast a pumpkin, cut it in half lengthways and scrape out the seeds. Brush each half with coconut oil and season with 1 teaspoon of sea salt. Place the pumpkin halves with the cut side up on a baking tray and roast in the preheated oven for about 50 minutes, or until tender to the fork.

Ingredients:
- ✓ ½ teaspoon of red pepper flakes
- ✓ 1 (6-ounce / 170-g) can of tomato paste
- ✓ 1 (16-ounce / 454-g) jar of spaghetti sauce
- ✓ ½ cup of water

- ❖ In a medium saucepan over medium heat, add the onion and coconut oil. Fry for about 5 minutes, or until tender.
- ❖ Add the remaining salt, garlic, red pepper flakes and tomato paste. Stir until just combined.
- ❖ Add the spaghetti sauce and water. Cook on a low heat for 10 minutes.
- ❖ Add the spaghetti to the pumpkin and stir to combine.
- ❖ Serve immediately.

32) Peppers stuffed with vegetables and quinoa

Preparation time: 5 minutes **Cooking time**: 20 minutes **Portions**: 2

Ingredients:
- ✓ Cooking spray
- ✓ 1 teaspoon of coconut oil
- ✓ ½ cup of chopped vegetables, courgettes, carrots or broccoli
- ✓ 1 cup of cooked quinoa

Directions:
- ❖ Preheat the oven to 350°F (180°C).
- ❖ Coat a baking tray with cooking spray.
- ❖ In a medium saucepan over medium heat, add the coconut oil and chopped vegetables. Fry for 5 minutes, or until softened.
- ❖ Add the quinoa, garlic powder, onion powder and salt. Stir to combine.

Ingredients:
- ✓ 1 teaspoon of garlic powder
- ✓ 1 teaspoon onion powder
- ✓ 1 teaspoon sea salt
- ✓ 2 peppers, any colour, with core and seeds; the tops have been removed and reserved

- ❖ Place each pepper upright in the prepared baking tray. Fill each pepper with half of the quinoa and vegetable mix. Cover each pepper with its reserved top.
- ❖ Cover with aluminium foil, place in the preheated oven and bake for 15 minutes, or until the peppers are soft.

33) Aubergine curry with quinoa

Preparation time: 5 minutes **Cooking time**: 35 minutes **Portions**: 2

Ingredients:
- ✓ 1 aubergine, cooled, with contents removed from the shell and reserved
- ✓ Juice of 1 lemon
- ✓ 1 teaspoon sea salt
- ✓ 1 teaspoon of sesame oil

Directions:
- ❖ Preheat the oven to 300°F.
- ❖ To roast aubergines, simply slice them, add a little sea salt and cook them in the preheated oven for about 30 minutes, or until soft.
- ❖ In a food processor, combine the aubergine, lemon juice, salt, sesame oil and curry powder. Blend until smooth.

Ingredients:
- ✓ 1 teaspoon curry powder
- ✓ Water, as required
- ✓ Cooked quinoa, to serve

- ❖ In a small saucepan over medium heat, transfer the aubergine mixture and heat it for about 5 minutes. Add a little water to dilute, if necessary.
- ❖ Serve on top of the quinoa.

34) Chili with barbecue bean sauce

Preparation time: 5 minutes **Cooking time:** 25 minutes **Portions: 4**

Ingredients:
- ✓ Cooking spray
- ✓ 1 small onion, chopped
- ✓ 1 cup diced red pepper
- ✓ 2 cloves of garlic, finely chopped
- ✓ 2 cups of sprouted black, kidney or pinto beans
- ✓ 1 (14.5-ounce / 411-g) can of diced tomatoes

Directions:
- ❖ Spray a medium-sized saucepan with cooking spray. Put it over a medium heat. Add the onions and fry for 5 minutes, or until soft and slightly caramelised.

Ingredients:
- ✓ 2 tablespoons of barbecue sauce
- ✓ 1 (8-ounce / 227-g) jar of organic pasta sauce
- ✓ ¼ cup organic sauce, sweet, medium or hot
- ✓ ¼ cup fresh organic coriander
- ✓ A pinch of chilli powder
- ✓ A pinch of ground cumin

- ❖ Add the pepper, garlic, sprouted beans, tomatoes, homemade barbecue sauce, pasta sauce, salsa, cilantro, chilli powder and cumin. Stir to combine. Cook over a low heat for 20 minutes.
- ❖ Serve immediately.

35) Cooking broccoli and carrots

Preparation time: 10 minutes **Cooking time:** 30 minutes **Portions: 2**

Ingredients:
- ✓ 1 lb (454 g) broccoli, chopped
- ✓ 4 carrots, peeled and sliced
- ✓ 3 garlic heads, cloves peeled and chopped, or 3 tablespoons chopped
- ✓ 2 teaspoons of lemon peel

Directions:
- ❖ Preheat the oven to 400°F (205°C).
- ❖ In a medium bowl, mix together the broccoli, carrots, garlic, lemon zest, salt, mustard powder, stock and coconut oil.

Ingredients:
- ✓ 1 teaspoon sea salt
- ✓ ¼ teaspoon mustard powder
- ✓ 1 cup of vegetable stock
- ✓ 2 tablespoons of coconut oil

- ❖ Spread the mixture evenly in the baking tin. Cover with aluminium foil and place in the preheated oven. Bake for 30 minutes, stirring once.
- ❖ Serve immediately.

36) Ratatouille

Preparation time: 15 minutes **Cooking time:** 35 minutes **Portions: 4**

Ingredients:
- ✓ Cooking spray
- ✓ ½ onion, chopped
- ✓ 2 cloves of garlic, minced
- ✓ 1 (6-ounce / 170-g) can of tomato paste
- ✓ 4 tablespoons of coconut oil, divided by
- ✓ ¾ cup of water
- ✓ ½ teaspoon of sea salt
- ✓ 1 small aubergine, thinly sliced

Directions:
- ❖ Preheat the oven to 375°F (190°C).
- ❖ Spray a small frying pan with cooking spray. Put the pan over medium heat, add the onion and garlic and fry for 5 minutes, or until soft. Remove from heat and set aside.
- ❖ In a small bowl, combine the tomato paste, onion mixture, 1 tablespoon of coconut oil and the water. Season with salt. Spread this mixture over the bottom of a baking dish.
- ❖ In a large bowl, add the aubergines, courgettes, yellow squash, red pepper, yellow pepper, tomatoes and 1 tablespoon of coconut oil. Stir to evenly coat all the vegetables.

Ingredients:
- ✓ 1 courgette, thinly sliced
- ✓ 1 yellow pumpkin, thinly sliced
- ✓ 1 red pepper, thinly sliced
- ✓ 1 yellow pepper, thinly sliced
- ✓ 2 large tomatoes, thinly sliced
- ✓ 1 teaspoon of fresh thyme leaves

- ❖ Following the inside edge of the baking tray and working inwards, cover the tomato mixture with the vegetables, layering and alternating by type (e.g. 1 slice of aubergine, then 1 slice of courgette, 1 slice of pumpkin, 1 slice of red pepper, 1 slice of yellow pepper, and finally, 1 slice of tomato). Repeat the layers in a spiral until all the vegetables are used.
- ❖ Season with thyme and finish by drizzling the remaining 2 tablespoons of coconut oil over the vegetables. Cover with aluminium foil, or parchment paper, and place in the preheated oven.
- ❖ Cook for about 30 minutes, or until the vegetables are tender and fully roasted.

37) Fruit and vegetable roast Ritzy

Preparation time: 15 minutes **Cooking time**: 60 minutes **Portions**: 4

Ingredients:
- 1 butternut squash, peeled and diced
- 1 baked pumpkin, peeled and diced
- 2 large carrots, peeled and diced
- 2 green apples, peeled, cored and sliced

Directions:
- Preheat the oven to 350ºF (180ºC).
- In a large bowl, combine the pumpkin, squash, carrots, apples, sage, salt and coconut oil.

Ingredients:
- 3 fresh sage leaves, finely chopped
- 1 teaspoon sea salt
- 2 teaspoons of coconut oil

- Stir to evenly coat the oil and seasonings. Transfer the vegetables to an ovenproof dish, in a single layer.
- Roast for 60 minutes, stirring occasionally. Serve.

38) Brussels sprouts with coconut

Preparation time: 5 minutes **Cooking time**: 10 minutes **Portions**: 2

Ingredients:
- ½ cup of light unsweetened coconut milk
- 1 teaspoon freshly squeezed lime juice
- 1½ teaspoons of ground ginger
- ½ teaspoon of chilli and garlic sauce

Directions:
- In a medium saucepan over medium heat, combine the coconut milk, lime juice, ground ginger, chilli and garlic sauce and stevia. Bring the ingredients to the boil. Cook for 5 minutes. Remove from the heat and set aside.
- Preheat the grill.
- In a medium bowl, add the Brussels sprouts, coconut oil and sea salt. Stir to combine.

Ingredients:
- 1 packet of stevia
- ¾ of a pound (340 g) of Brussels sprouts, without ends, cut and halved
- 1 tablespoon of coconut oil
- ½ teaspoon of sea salt

- Transfer to a medium cast-iron skillet or ovenproof pan. Fry over a medium heat for 5 minutes.
- Place the pan under the grill and cook for 3 minutes, or until the leaves are lightly browned.
- Transfer the Brussels sprouts to a medium bowl. Add the sauce and stir to coat. Serve immediately.

39) Pasta with basil spinach pesto

Preparation time: 10 minutes **Cooking time**: 10 minutes **Portions**: 4

Ingredients:
- 2 cups gluten-free dried pasta
- 3 cups of packed spinach
- ½ cup packed fresh basil
- 3 tablespoons avocado oil

Directions:
- Bring a pot of water to the boil and cook the pasta according to the package instructions. Drain, transfer to a large bowl and set aside.

Ingredients:
- 3 tablespoons of walnut pieces
- 1 or 2 garlic cloves, peeled
- ⅛ teaspoon of sea salt

- In a food processor, combine the spinach, basil, oil, walnuts, garlic and salt and pulse for 20-30 seconds until the desired consistency is reached. Mix the pesto with the cooked pasta and serve.

40) Mushroom and onion risotto

Preparation time: 5 minutes **Cooking time:** 1 hour 25 minutes **Portions: 2**

Ingredients:
- ✓ 4 ounces (113 g) sliced mushrooms
- ✓ ¼ chopped onion
- ✓ 1 cup of wild rice
- ✓ 1 tablespoon of grape oil

Ingredients:
- ✓ 2 cups of home-made vegetable broth
- ✓ ⅓ teaspoon of salt
- ✓ ¼ teaspoon cayenne pepper

Directions:
- ❖ Take a medium saucepan, put it on a medium heat, add the oil and when it is hot, add the onion and mushrooms and then cook for 4 to 5 minutes until the mushrooms have turned golden and the liquid in the pan has evaporated.
- ❖ Add rice, stir until combined, cook for 1 minute, then stir in salt and cayenne pepper.
- ❖ Pour in the stock, lower the heat and cook the rice for 1 hour and 20 minutes until tender.
- ❖ Serve immediately.

41) Vegetable bowl with basil and quinoa

Preparation time: 5 minutes **Cooking time:** 3 minutes **Portions: 2**

Ingredients:
- ✓ ⅓ cup of quinoa, cooked
- ✓ ¼ cup cherry tomatoes, quartered
- ✓ ½ green pepper, chopped
- ✓ ⅓ cup of basil leaves

Ingredients:
- ✓ 1 tablespoon of grape oil
- ✓ ¼ teaspoon of salt
- ✓ ⅛ teaspoon of cayenne pepper

Directions:
- ❖ Take a frying pan, put it on a medium heat, add the oil and when it is hot, add the cherry tomatoes and the pepper and cook for 2 to 3 minutes until they are tender and crispy.
- ❖ Take a medium bowl, put the cooked quinoa in it, add the tomato and pepper mixture and then add the basil leaves.
- ❖ Season with salt and cayenne pepper, stir until combined, then serve.

42) Spelt sultana biscuits

Preparation time: 10 minutes **Cooking time:** 18 minutes **Portions: 2**

Ingredients:
- ✓ 1 cup of spelt flour
- ✓ ⅓ cup of sultanas
- ✓ ½ cup of pitted dates
- ✓ 3½ tablespoons of homemade apple sauce or apple puree

Ingredients:
- ✓ ⅔ tablespoon of spring water
- ✓ ¹⁄₁₆ teaspoon of sea salt
- ✓ 2 tablespoons agave syrup
- ✓ 1 ¾ tablespoons of grape oil

Directions:
- ❖ Turn on the oven, then set it to 350°F (180°C) and let it preheat.
- ❖ Meanwhile, place the flour in a food processor, add the dates and salt, and then pulse until well combined.
- ❖ Transfer the flour mixture to a medium bowl, add the remaining ingredients and stir until well mixed.
- ❖ Divide the dough into parts, each part about 2 tablespoons, and then shape each part into a ball.
- ❖ Place the biscuit ball on a baking tray lined with baking paper, flatten it slightly with a fork and then bake for 18 minutes until cooked through.
- ❖ Let the biscuits cool down for 10 minutes and then serve.

43) Quinoa and chickpea burgers

Preparation time: 10 minutes   **Cooking time**: 20 minutes   **Portions**: 2

Ingredients:
- ✓ 2 tablespoons chopped onion
- ✓ ¾ cup of chickpeas
- ✓ ¼ cup of cooked quinoa
- ✓ 1 tablespoon of spring water

Directions:
- ❖ Turn on the oven, then set it to 375°F (190°C) and let it preheat.
- ❖ Meanwhile, put the onion, chickpeas and quinoa in a food processor and then give a small pulse to make a chunky mixture.
- ❖ Add the water, salt and cayenne pepper and then pulse until the mixture comes together.
- ❖ Then pour the mixture into a medium bowl, cover it with its lid and then leave it to rest in the fridge for 15 minutes.

Ingredients:
- ✓ 1 tablespoon of grape oil
- ✓ ⅓ teaspoon of salt
- ✓ ¼ teaspoon cayenne pepper

- ❖ Form the mixture into two patties, place them on a baking tray lined with baking paper and then bake for 20 minutes, turning halfway through.
- ❖ Then turn on the grill and continue cooking for 2 minutes per side until golden brown.
- ❖ You can serve the patties with spelt flour burgers and tahini butter.

44) Chickpea burgers with teff

Preparation time: 10 minutes   **Cooking time**: 8 minutes   **Portions**: 2

Ingredients:
- ✓ ¾ cup of cooked teff grains
- ✓ ¾ cup of chickpea flour
- ✓ 2 tablespoons diced onion
- ✓ 2 tablespoons diced red peppers
- ✓ ½ teaspoon of dill

Directions:
- ❖ Take a medium-sized frying pan, place it over a medium heat, add the oil and when it is hot, add the onion and pepper and cook for 3 minutes until tender.
- ❖ Transfer the vegetables to a large bowl, add the remaining ingredients, mix until combined, and then shape the mixture into meatballs.

Ingredients:
- ✓ ¼ teaspoon of salt
- ✓ ½ teaspoon of oregano
- ✓ ⅛ teaspoon of cayenne pepper
- ✓ ½ teaspoon of basil
- ✓ 1 tablespoon of grape oil

- ❖ Place the meatballs in the pan and then cook for 3 minutes per side until they are crispy and golden brown on all sides.
- ❖ Serve immediately.

45) Kamut nut porridge

Preparation time: 5 minutes   **Cooking time**: 10 minutes   **Portions**: 2

Ingredients:
- ✓ ½ cup kamut
- ✓ ¼ teaspoon of salt
- ✓ 2 tablespoons agave syrup

Directions:
- ❖ Plug in a high-speed food processor or blender, add the kamut to its jar and then pulse until it splits.
- ❖ Take a medium saucepan, add the kamut together with the salt, pour in the milk and then stir until combined.

Ingredients:
- ✓ ½ tablespoon of coconut oil
- ✓ 2 cups of home-made nut milk

- ❖ Place the saucepan over high heat, bring the mixture to the boil, then lower the heat to medium-low and simmer for 5-10 minutes until it has thickened to the desired level.
- ❖ Then remove the pan from the heat, mix the agave syrup and oil into the oatmeal and then distribute evenly between two bowls.
- ❖ Garnish the oatmeal with fruit approved by Dr Sebi's Diet and then serve.

46) Blueberry, banana and amaranth pancakes

Preparation time: 10 minutes **Cooking time:** 6 minutes **Portions:** 2

Ingredients:
- ½ cup of chickpea flour
- ¼ cup blueberries
- 1 butter banana, peeled
- ½ cup amaranth greens
- ½ cup of spring water

Directions:
- Plug in a food processor or high-speed blender and add all the ingredients into its jar.
- Cover the blender jar with its lid, pulse for 40-60 seconds until smooth, pour the mixture into a bowl and let it rest for 10 minutes.

Ingredients:
- ½ teaspoon of sea salt
- 1 tablespoon agave syrup
- 1 tablespoon nut butter
- 1 tablespoon of grape oil

- When you're ready to cook, take a large frying pan, place it over medium-high heat, add the oil and then let it heat up.
- Pour the prepared batter into the hot pan in six portions, shape each portion like a pancake and then cook for 2 to 3 minutes per side until the edges are cooked and firm.
- Serve immediately.

47) Chickpea meatloaf with mushrooms and pepper

Preparation time: 10 minutes **Cooking time:** 45 minutes **Portions:** 2

Ingredients:
- ¼ cup of spelt flour
- 1½ cups chickpeas, cooked
- ¾ cup of diced onions
- ¼ cup chopped basil
- ½ cup sliced white mushrooms
- 1 red pepper, core, diced
- 1 tablespoon of grape oil

Directions:
- Turn on the oven, then set it to 350°F (180°C) and let it preheat.
- In the meantime, take a large frying pan, put it over medium-high heat, add the oil and when it is hot, add the onion, pepper and mushrooms and then cook for 3 minutes or until they start to become tender.
- Add the chopped basil to the pan, stir until combined, remove the pan from the heat, add all the seasonings and then stir until combined.

Ingredients:
- 1 ¼ teaspoons of granulated onion, homemade
- ⅛ teaspoon dried thyme
- ½ teaspoon of sea salt and more if necessary
- ⅓ teaspoon of dried sage
- ¼ teaspoon of cayenne pepper and more if necessary
- ¼ teaspoon dried oregano

- Place the chickpeas in a food processor, pulse until coarsely chopped, then transfer to a medium bowl.
- Add the cooked vegetable mixture together with the remaining ingredients, mix until well combined and then spoon into a greased baking dish.
- Bake the loaf for 30-40 minutes until firm and cooked through, cool slightly, cut into slices and then serve.

48) Fried rice with mushrooms and courgettes

Preparation time: 5 minutes **Cooking time:** 15 minutes **Portions:** 2

Ingredients:
- ½ cup of sliced mushrooms
- 1 cup cooked wild rice
- ½ cup of sliced red pepper
- ¼ of a medium-sized onion, peeled and diced

Directions:
- Take a medium frying pan, put it over medium heat, add the oil and when it is hot, add the onion and cook for 5 minutes until browned.
- Add the remaining vegetables, stir until combined, and then cook for 5 minutes until almost soft.

Ingredients:
- ½ cup of sliced courgettes
- ½ teaspoon of salt
- ¼ teaspoon cayenne pepper
- 1 tablespoon of grape oil

- Add the rice, stir until combined and cook for 3 minutes until golden brown.
- Serve immediately.

49) Kamut and date porridge

Preparation time: 5 minutes **Cooking time:** 15 minutes **Portions:** 2

Ingredients:
- 1 cup of dates, pitted, chopped
- 1 cup rolled kamut flakes

Ingredients:
- ⅛ teaspoon of salt
- 2 cups of spring water

Directions:
- Put the kamut flakes in a small saucepan, pour in the water and leave to soak overnight.
- Then, stir in the salt, place the pan over medium-high heat and bring the mixture to a simmer.
- Change the heat to medium-low and continue cooking for 10 minutes or more until all the liquid has been absorbed.
- Remove the pan from the heat, add the dates to the oatmeal and then stir until mixed.
- Divide the oatmeal between two bowls, drizzle with agave syrup if necessary and then serve.

50) Blackberry-flavoured banana and quinoa bars

Preparation time: 10 minutes **Cooking time:** 10 minutes **Portions:** 2

Ingredients:
- ½ cup of spelt flour
- 2 bananas child butter
- 1 cup quinoa flakes
- ¹⁄₁₆ teaspoon of sea salt

Ingredients:
- 1 tablespoon agave nectar
- ¼ cup of grape oil
- ½ cup of alkaline blackberry jam

Directions:
- Turn on the oven, then set it to 350°F (180°C) and let it preheat.
- Meanwhile, place the bananas, peeled from the butter, in a medium bowl and then mash them with a fork.
- Add the agave nectar and oil, mix until well combined, and then stir in the salt, flour and quinoa flakes until you have a sticky dough.
- Take a square dish, line it with a sheet of parchment, spread two-thirds of the prepared pastry on the bottom, layer with the blackberry jam and then cover with the remaining pastry.
- Bake for 10 minutes and then leave the mixture to cool for 15 minutes.
- Cut the dough into 4 bars and then serve.

51) Amaranth and courgette meatballs

Preparation time: 10 minutes **Cooking time:** 12 minutes **Portions:** 2

Ingredients:
- ½ cup amaranth, cooked
- ½ medium white onion, peeled, chopped
- ¼ cup grated courgettes
- ¼ cup chopped red pepper
- ⅓ teaspoon of salt

Ingredients:
- ¼ teaspoon cayenne pepper
- ¼ teaspoon of coriander powder
- ¼ teaspoon of key lime zest
- 2 tablespoons of grape oil

Directions:
- Take a small frying pan, put it over medium heat, add 1 tablespoon of oil and when it is hot, add the onion and then cook for 5 minutes until tender.
- Add the courgettes and red pepper, stir until combined and cook for 3 minutes.
- Add the remaining ingredients except the oil and amaranth, stir until combined, then remove the pan from the heat and cool for 10 minutes.
- Take a medium bowl, place the cooked amaranth in it, add the vegetable mixture, stir until combined, and then form into evenly sized patties.
- Take a large frying pan, place over a medium heat, add the remaining oil and when hot, place the meatballs in it and then cook for 3 minutes on each side until golden brown.
- Serve immediately.

52) Spiced chickpeas and cherry tomatoes

Preparation time: 5 minutes   **Cooking time:** 10 minutes   **Portions:** 2

Ingredients:
- ½ cup of cooked chickpeas
- 8 cherry tomatoes, chopped
- 1 medium onion, peeled, sliced
- ¾ cup of home-made vegetable broth
- 6 teaspoons of spice mixture

Ingredients:
- ¼ teaspoon of salt
- ½ tablespoon of grape oil
- ¼ teaspoon cayenne pepper
- ¾ cup of tomato sauce, alkaline
- 6 tablespoons of soft coconut milk jelly

Directions:
- Take a large frying pan, put it over medium heat, add the oil and heat, add the onion, and then cook for 5 minutes until golden brown.
- Add the spice mix, add the remaining ingredients to the pan except the okra, stir until combined, and then bring the mixture to a simmer.
- Add the chickpeas, stir until combined, and then cook for 5 minutes over medium-low heat until fully heated.
- Serve immediately.

53) Herb rice bowl

Preparation time: 5 minutes   **Cooking time:** 45 minutes   **Portions:** 2

Ingredients:
- 1 cup of wild rice
- ½ teaspoon dried basil
- ½ teaspoon dried thyme

Ingredients:
- ½ teaspoon dried oregano
- 3 cups of homemade vegetable broth
- ½ teaspoon of salt

Directions:
- Take a medium saucepan, place it over a medium-high heat, add the rice, pour in the water and bring it to the boil, covering the saucepan with a lid.
- Then turn the heat down to low and simmer the rice for 40 minutes until tender.
- Drain the excess liquid from the rice, add the herbs, stir until combined, and then serve.

54) Polenta with amaranth milk and walnuts

Preparation time: 5 minutes   **Cooking time:** 15 minutes   **Portions:** 2

Ingredients:
- ¾ cup amaranth
- ¼ teaspoon of onion powder
- ¼ teaspoon of salt

Ingredients:
- 6 tablespoons of homemade nut milk
- 1½ cups of home-made vegetable stock
- ⅛ teaspoon of cayenne pepper

Directions:
- Take a medium saucepan, place it over medium heat, pour in the stock, stir in the salt and then bring it to the boil.
- Then change the heat to medium-low, whisk in the amaranth and cook for 10-20 minutes until the mixture is slightly thick.
- Add the remaining ingredients, stir until combined, and continue cooking for 5 minutes.
- Serve the polenta with chickpeas.

55) Breaded peppers with walnuts

Preparation time: 5 minutes   **Cooking time:** 15 minutes   **Portions:** 2

Ingredients:
- 8 ounces (227 g) walnuts, soaked overnight
- ¼ cup of sliced green peppers
- ½ cup of sliced white onions
- ¼ cup sliced red peppers
- ¼ cup of sliced orange peppers
- 1 tablespoon onion powder

Ingredients:
- ½ teaspoon of sea salt
- 1 teaspoon dried oregano
- ¼ teaspoon cayenne pepper
- 1 teaspoon dried basil
- 2 tablespoons of grape oil
- 2 tablespoons of spring water

Directions:
- Drain the walnuts, place them in a food processor and pulse them until they become crumbs.
- Take a frying pan, put it over medium-high heat, add the oil and when it is hot, add the onions and all the peppers, toss with all the seasonings and then cook for 10 minutes until tender.
- Add the walnuts, stir in the water and cook for 3 to 5 minutes until hot.
- Serve hot.

56) Pumpkin and amaranth bowl

Preparation time: 5 minutes **Cooking time:** 10 minutes **Portions:** 2

Ingredients:
- ✓ 10 ounces (283 g) of cooked butternut squash chunks
- ✓ 1 apple, peeled, pitted, sliced
- ✓ 8 ounces (227 g) of green cabbage
- ✓ 1 teaspoon garam masala

Directions:
- ❖ Take a frying pan, put it on a medium heat, add 1 teaspoon of oil and when it is hot, add the pumpkin piece, sprinkle with the garam masala and ¼ teaspoon of salt, stir until combined and then cook for 5 minutes until hot.

Ingredients:
- ✓ 1½ cups cooked amaranth
- ✓ ½ teaspoon of salt
- ✓ ¼ teaspoon cayenne pepper
- ✓ 1 teaspoon and 1 tablespoon of grape oil
- ❖ Transfer the pumpkin mixture to a bowl, return the pan to medium heat, add the remaining oil, and when hot, add the cabbage tops, season with the remaining salt, and then cook for 5 minutes until hot.
- ❖ Divide the amaranth between two bowls, add the apple, collard and pumpkin mixture and serve.

57) Chickpea and veg hot dogs

Preparation time: 5 minutes **Cooking time:** 10 minutes **Portions:** 2

Ingredients:
- ✓ 1 cup of cooked chickpeas
- ✓ ⅓ cup of diced green pepper,
- ✓ 1 cup of spelt flour
- ✓ ⅓ cup of diced white onion,
- ✓ 1 teaspoon of coriander
- ✓ ¼ cup diced shallots,

Directions:
- ❖ Take a frying pan, put it on a medium heat, add the oil and when it is hot, add the chickpeas and all the vegetables and cook for 5 minutes.
- ❖ Transfer the chickpeas and vegetables to a food processor, add the remaining ingredients and pulse until well combined.
- ❖ Shape the mixture into hot dog-shaped rolls, and then wrap each hot dog in baking paper.

Ingredients:
- ✓ 1 tablespoon onion powder
- ✓ 2 teaspoons of sea salt
- ✓ ½ teaspoon of dill
- ✓ 1 tablespoon of grape oil
- ✓ ½ cup of chickpea liquid

- ❖ Boil some water in a pot, put a steamer on it, put the wrapped hot dogs on it and then steam for 30 minutes.
- ❖ Once done, uncover the hot dogs and then fry them for 10 minutes over medium heat until golden brown on all sides.
- ❖ Serve the hot dogs in spelt buns.

DINNER

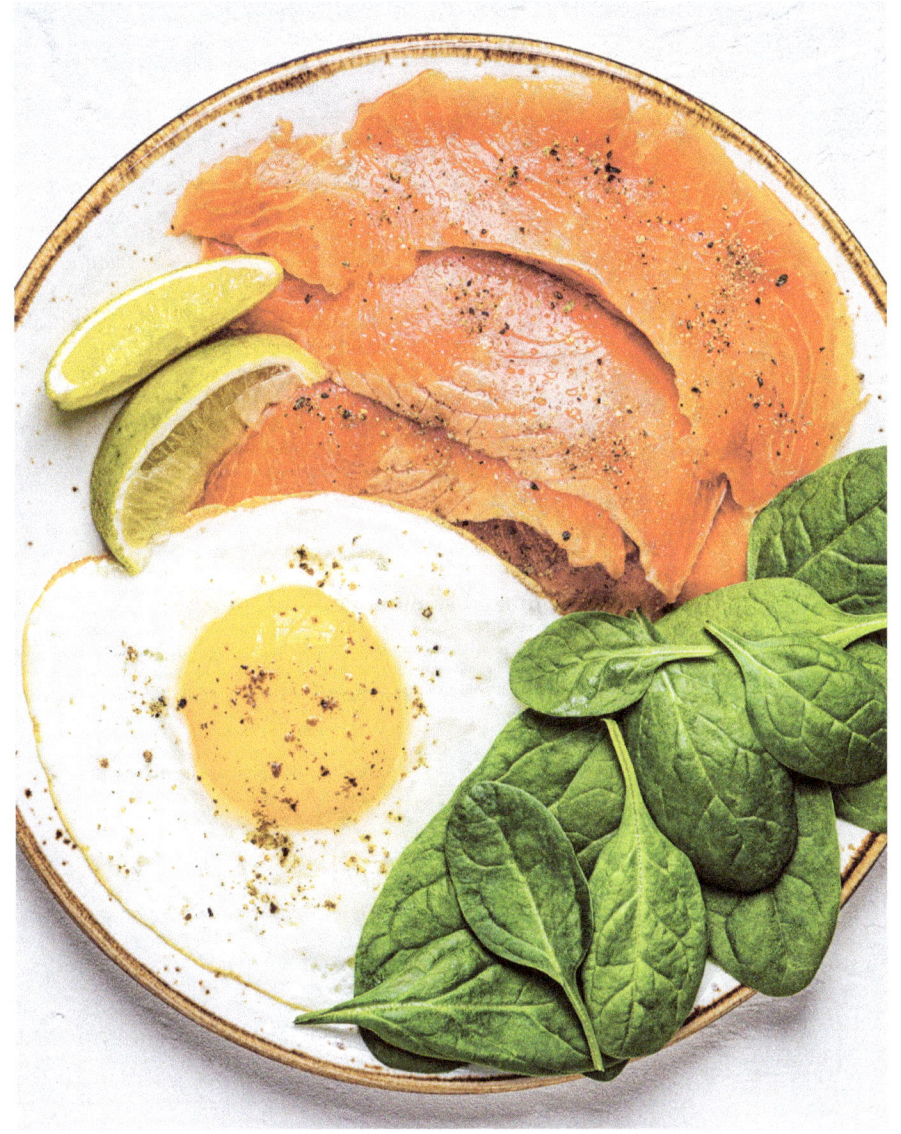

58) Sesame and quinoa pilaf

Preparation time: **Cooking time:** **Portions:**

Ingredients:
- ✓ Cooked green lentils (1 c.)
- ✓ Broth or water (1 c.)
- ✓ Quinoa (.5 c.)
- ✓ Chopped garlic clove (1)
- ✓ Diced green pepper (.5 c.)
- ✓ Celery stalk, diced (1)
- ✓ Sliced shallot (1)
- ✓ Crushed pepper (2 teaspoons)
- ✓ Salt (2 teaspoons)
- ✓ Olive oil (2 tablespoons)
- ✓ Sliced carrots (2)

Ingredients:
- ✓ Green beans cut and sliced (1 c.)
- ✓ For the dressing
- ✓ Black sesame seeds (2 tablespoons)
- ✓ Rice vinegar (.25 c.)
- ✓ Tamari (.25 c.)
- ✓ Red pepper flakes (.5 tsp.)
- ✓ Lemon peel (1 teaspoon)
- ✓ Grated ginger (1 teaspoon)
- ✓ Toasted sesame oil (2 tablespoons)
- ✓ Avocado oil (.33 c.)

Directions:
- ❖ Place the carrots and green beans on baking paper on a baking tray. Sprinkle with pepper, salt and a tablespoon of olive oil.
- ❖ Add to the grill of the oven and bake until golden brown. This will take about five minutes.
- ❖ Once this is done, take a pot and add the garlic, pepper, celery, shallot and the rest of the oil.
- ❖ Cook the ingredients for five minutes before adding the quinoa and stirring to cook a little longer.
- ❖ Now add the water or broth and bring to the boil. Let it simmer for a while until the liquid has disappeared.
- ❖ Now you can prepare the dressing. To do this, whisk all the ingredients in a bowl to combine them.
- ❖ When it's time to assemble, mix together the quinoa and lentils. Season with a little pepper and salt and then add the carrot and bean mixture before pouring the dressing over everything.

59) Smoked salmon with fruit sauce

Preparation time: **Cooking time:** **Portions:**

Ingredients:
- ✓ Mixed vegetables (4 c.)
- ✓ Olive oil (1 tablespoon)
- ✓ Crushed pepper (.25 tsp.)
- ✓ Salt (.25 tsp.)
- ✓ Chilli powder (.5 tsp.)
- ✓ Garlic powder (1 teaspoon)
- ✓ Cayenne pepper (1 teaspoon)
- ✓ Salmon (8 oz)

Ingredients:
- ✓ To make the sauce
- ✓ Halls
- ✓ Chopped coriander (1 tablespoon)
- ✓ Lime juice and zest (1)
- ✓ Diced pineapple (.5 c.)
- ✓ Diced mango (.5 c.)
- ✓ Diced green pepper (.5)

Directions:
- ❖ Start this recipe by preparing the mango and pineapple salsa. Add all the ingredients to a bowl and stir to combine. Set aside for now.
- ❖ In another bowl, combine together the pepper, salt, chilli powder, garlic powder and cayenne. Place this mixture on a flat plate to use at the appropriate time.
- ❖ Heat a frying pan on the cooker over medium heat. Brush olive oil all over the salmon fillet before adding the meat side to the spice mixture on the pan.
- ❖ Add the meat side to the pan and let it cook. After five minutes, turn the fish over and cook a little longer until the fish is done.
- ❖ Serve the fish with the chosen mixed vegetables and a little sauce on top.

60) Rocket salad with shrimps

Preparation time: **Cooking time:** **Portions:**

Ingredients:
- Crushed black pepper (.5 tsp.)
- Salt (.5 tsp.)
- Chopped parsley (1 tablespoon)
- Chopped garlic clove (1)
- Olive oil (2 tablespoons)
- Lemon juice (.5)
- Prawn (10)
- For the salad

Ingredients:
- Toasted pine nuts (2 tablespoons)
- Salt (1 teaspoon)
- Olive oil (2 tablespoons)
- Lemon juice (.5)
- Apple cider vinegar (2 tablespoons)
- Halved cherry tomatoes (10)
- Rocket (4 c.)

Directions:
- Take out a bowl and add the pepper, parsley, salt, garlic, olive oil, lemon juice and prawns. Place in the fridge to marinate for fifteen minutes or more.
- When you are ready, take out a frying pan and heat it up. Add the prepared prawns to the inside and cook a little on each side until the prawns are all cooked.
- Now it is time to prepare the salad. Take out a large salad bowl and combine all the salad ingredients.
- Add the prawns on top of the salad and serve hot.

61) Easy pizza

Preparation time: **Cooking time:** **Portions:**

Ingredients:
- Lemon juice (1 teaspoon)
- Salt (1 teaspoon)
- Nutritional yeast (2 tablespoons)
- Olive oil (2 tablespoons)
- Rocket (1c)
- Sliced tomato (1)
- Sliced avocado (1)
- For the pasta
- Dried basil (1 teaspoon)

Ingredients:
- Dried oregano (1 teaspoon)
- Pepper (1 teaspoon)
- Salt (1 teaspoon)
- Olive oil (4 tablespoons)
- Chopped garlic clove (1)
- Ground linseed (.33 c.)
- Sunflower seeds, soaked (1.25 c.)

Directions:
- Take out a blender and blend the sunflower seeds a couple of times. Then add them to a large bowl along with the basil, oregano, salt, pepper, olive oil, garlic and flaxseed meal.
- Knead this mixture until it forms a good dough. More water can be added if necessary.
- Roll out the dough into a pizza shape. Place some baking paper on your baking tray and place the dough on top.
- Heat your oven to the lowest possible temperature and then place the tray inside to dehydrate the dough. Give it about 12 hours to finish.
- When the dough is ready, you can put the tomato slices and avocado on top of the crust.
- Chop the rocket in a small bowl with the lemon juice, salt, nutritional yeast and olive oil. Place this on top of the pizza and serve immediately.

62) Spelt bread

Preparation time: **Cooking time:** **Portions:**

Ingredients:
- 3/4 - 1 cup alkaline water
- ½ cup unsweetened hemp milk
- 3 tablespoons avocado oil

Directions:
- Preheat the oven to 375 degrees F. Meanwhile, combine all the dry contents in a bowl.
- Add ¾ cup of water, the hemp milk and the avocado oil until completely blended to create a smooth batter.
- If the batter seems rather stiff, add a few tablespoons of alkaline water until the dough is soft. And if it's too wet, add a few more tablespoons of spelt flour, stirring after each spoonful until the batter holds together well.
- Cover the work surface with about ½ cup of spelt flour. Then knead the dough on the floured surface and roll it to coat it with flour.
- Knead the dough for a further 2 to 3 minutes, and add a little more spelt with each addition until you have a unified ball that can go back when prodded.

Ingredients:
- 1 tablespoon agave nectar
- 1 ½ teaspoons of fine sea salt
- 4 cups spelt flour + ½ cup extra for kneading

- Now, take a baking paper and line a standard baking tray across its width. Take some avocado oil and grease the ends of the baking tray.
- Turn the dough into the prepared pan and pat it to distribute it well in the pan. Score the top of the loaf using a sharp knife, lengthways.
- Finally, bake the bread until cooked through, or for about 45 minutes.
- Remove from the oven and insert a toothpick into the centre of the bread. If the toothpick or a thin, sharp knife does not come out clean, bake for another 5-10 minutes.
- Let the loaf cool completely in the baking tray and then cut it into slices. Serve it with some soup and cover it with the avocado. Sprinkle also with smoked paprika and lemon if you like.

63) Green Goddess Bowl with Avocado Dressing

Preparation time: **Cooking time:** **Portions: 4**

Ingredients:
- For the salad:
- 2 tablespoons of hemp seeds
- 1/3 cup cherry tomatoes, halved
- ½ cup of kelp noodles, soaked and drained
- ½ courgette
- 3 cups of cabbage, chopped
- Avocado dressing:
- A pinch of cayenne pepper
- 1 tablespoon extra virgin olive oil
- ¼ teaspoon of sea salt
- 1 cup of filtered water

Directions:
- First make the courgette noodles using a spiralizer.
- Then lightly steam the cabbage for about 4 minutes and set aside.
- Combine the kelp noodles with the courgette noodles and toss together with the avocado and cumin seasoning.

Ingredients:
- 2 limes, freshly squeezed
- 1 tablespoon dried sage
- 1 avocado
- Tahini lemon dressing:
- 1 tablespoon extra virgin olive oil
- ¾ teaspoon of sea salt
- 1 fennel bulb
- ½ freshly squeezed lemon
- ½ cup of filtered water
- ¼ cup tahini, sesame butter
- Cayenne pepper to taste

- Now add the cherry tomatoes and mix well. Plate the steamed broccoli and cabbage and cover with the tahini dressing.
- Serve the cabbage with the tomatoes and noodles sprinkled with hemp seeds.

64) Asian sesame dressing and noodles

Preparation time: **Cooking time:** **Portions: 2**

Ingredients:
- 1 bag of Kelp Noodles or 1 courgette for making noodles
- 1 tablespoon raw sesame seeds, for garnish
- 1 shallot, chopped
- Parsnips, optional
- Sliced red pepper, optional

Directions:
- With a vegetable peeler or spiralizer, cut strips the size of a noodle or use 1 bag of kelp noodles.
- Mix all the ingredients for the seasoning in a bowl, and stir well with a spoon. If using kelp noodles, place them in hot water for about 10 minutes to soften them.

Ingredients:
- For the dressing:
- 1 fennel bulb, chopped
- ½ teaspoon lemon, freshly squeezed
- ½ teaspoon agave sugar
- 2 tablespoons of tahini, sesame butter

- Pour the sesame dressing over the scallions and noodles and mix well. Top with the sesame, if you like, and enjoy.

65) Instant alkaline sushi roll-up

Preparation time: **Cooking time:** **Portions: 2**

Ingredients:
For Dip/Hummus
- 1 fennel bulb
- A drop of olive oil
- 1 pinch of dried sage
- 1 tablespoon tahini
- A handful of walnuts
- 100 g canned chickpeas/garbanzos, drained
- Pinch of Himalayan salt
- Juice of 1/2 lemon

Directions:
- In a blender or food processor, blend all the ingredients for the hummus. Add a little lemon and olive oil in equal amounts until the desired consistency is achieved.
- To make the alkaline rolls, first cut the courgettes or pumpkin into long, thin strips with a vegetable peeler.

Ingredients:
For Roll-Ups
- 1 pepper cut into matchsticks
- 1 small bunch of culantro
- 1 avocado, peeled and sliced
- 1 cucumber, cut into matchsticks
- 1 parsnip, cut into matchsticks
- 2 medium-sized courgettes/courts

- Lay out the individual courgette strips and spread a generous amount of almond hummus on the courgette strip.
- Now add small amounts of avocado, strainer and vegetable matches.
- Add a few sesame seeds and serve.

66) Spaghetti filled with quinoa

Preparation time: **Cooking time:** **Portions: 2**

Ingredients:
- 1 teaspoon chopped ginger
- 2 teaspoons dried thyme
- 1 1/2 cups of cooked quinoa
- 1/4 cup chopped walnuts
- 2 spring onions, white part, sliced
- 1 orange or red pepper

Directions:
- Preheat the oven to 400 degrees F.
- Then clean the pumpkins, cut them in half and discard the seeds. Cook the pumpkins for about 40 minutes or until tender.
- In the meantime, in a frying pan, heat a tablespoon of coconut oil and cook the pepper and chopped shallots until soft.

Ingredients:
- 1 medium shallot
- 1 cup steamed green peas
- 2 tablespoons of coconut oil
- 1 large pumpkin or two smaller pumpkins
- Sea salt and cayenne pepper to taste

- Then add the cooked quinoa, green peas, spices and nuts and cook until heated through. Season the mixture with salt and pepper.
- Now divide the mixture between the pumpkins and cook until cooked through, or for about 5-8 minutes.
- Remove from the heat and serve the stuffed noodles with fresh vegetables such as cabbage.

67) Spelt pasta with spicy aubergine sauce

Preparation time: **Cooking time:** **Portions: 2**

Ingredients:
- A little cold-pressed extra virgin olive oil
- 1 pinch of cayenne pepper
- 1/2 teaspoon organic sea salt
- 1 handful of fresh basil
- 1 cup of vegetable stock
- 1 small chilli pepper

Directions:
- Cook the spelt pasta according to the instructions on the packet.
- In the meantime, cut the pepper and the aubergine into cubes and then cut the basil, the fennel bulb, the onion and the chilli into small pieces.
- In a frying pan, heat some olive oil and then fry the fennel bulb and onions for a few minutes.
- Add the pepper cubes and aubergines together with the chilli and cook for a further 2 to 3 minutes.

Ingredients:
- 1 fennel bulb
- 1 medium-sized onion
- 1 fresh red pepper
- 1 fresh aubergine
- 1 cup of spelt pasta

- Now dissolve the vegetable stock in 1 cup of alkaline water and add the mixture to the pan.
- Simmer the contents, stirring a few times, for about 10 minutes over low heat.
- Add the basil and season with a little pepper and salt. Spread the sauce over the spelt pasta and enjoy!

68) Sesame cabbage with chickpeas

Preparation time: Cooking time: Portions: 2

Ingredients:
- 1 tablespoon sesame oil
- 1 tablespoon sesame seeds
- 2 tablespoons of lemon juice
- 15 ounces of chickpea beans
- 1 fennel bulb, chopped

Ingredients:
- 1 bunch of green onions, thinly sliced
- 2 tablespoons of olive oil
- Salt to taste
- 1 bunch of cabbage

Directions:
- Start by cutting the cabbage. Tear the leaves from the stalk, roll them up and cut them into small pieces.
- Add some olive oil to a frying pan and then fry the green onions and fennel on a low heat for about 1 minute.
- Add the beans and fry for another 4 to 5 minutes. Add the cabbage, lemon juice and season with a little salt.
- Cook until the cabbage has reduced in size. Serve the cabbage, drizzle with a little sesame oil and a few sesame seeds.

69) Alkaline vegan meatloaf

Preparation time: Cooking time: Serves 1 loaf of bread

Ingredients:
- 1 cup of prepared wild rice
- 1/2 cup homemade tomato sauce, split
- 1/2 cup chopped yellow or white onion, split
- 1/2 cup chopped green pepper, split
- 1 shallot, roughly chopped
- 2 cups of mixed mushrooms, coarsely chopped
- 1/4 teaspoon cloves
- 1/2 teaspoon of ginger
- 1/2 teaspoon tarragon

Ingredients:
- 1 teaspoon of thyme
- 1 teaspoon of sage
- 1 tablespoon sea salt
- 1 tablespoon onion powder
- 1 cup chickpea or spelt flour
- 1.5 cups of breadcrumbs (spelt flour)
- 2 cups of cooked chickpeas
- Cayenne to taste

Directions:
- Clean and dry the wild rice as required. Also prepare the chickpeas and set them aside.
- Mix the chickpea or spelt flour with the breadcrumbs and set the mixture aside.
- Cut up the green peppers and onions and put half of them on the side.
- Now chop the shallots and mushrooms and add them to a food processor; together with the chickpeas, half the onion, half the green peppers and the spices.
- Pulse the mixture until it is completely incorporated. Then add 2 tablespoons of tomato sauce and the wild rice, and continue blending until you have a coarse paste.
- Move the mixture to a bowl large enough to accommodate the remaining flour, breadcrumbs, onion and green pepper. Mix until everything is combined.
- Now place the mixture in a greased baking dish and cover with the remaining tomato sauce.
- Bake in a preheated oven at 350 degrees F for about 60-70 minutes, keeping an eye on the top so it doesn't burn.
- Then remove from the oven and leave to cool for about 30 minutes. Serve with a little sauce and vegetables and enjoy.

70) Alkaline pizza crust

Preparation time: **Cooking time:**   **Portions: 4**

Ingredients:
- 1 cup of spring water
- 2 teaspoons of grape oil
- 2 teaspoons of agave
- 1 teaspoon sea salt
- 1 teaspoon of onion powder
- 1 1/2 cups of spelt flour
- 2 teaspoons of sesame seeds
- Gaskets (optional)
- 1 teaspoon of oregano

Ingredients:
- Cherry tomatoes
- Onions
- For the pizza sauce
- 1/2 teaspoon of oregano
- 1/2 teaspoon of sea salt
- 1/2 teaspoon onion powder
- 2 tablespoons chopped onion
- 1 avocado
- Pinch of basil

Directions:
- First, preheat the oven to 400 degrees F.
- In a medium-sized bowl, mix all the ingredients with ½ cup of water.
- Add more water in small amounts until the dough becomes a ball, or add more flour if the dough seems fluid.
- Coat a baking tray with oil and add a little flour to your hands.
- Now roll out the thick dough in the baking tin and brush the top with extra grape oil.
- With a fork, make a few holes in the dough and bake it in the preheated oven for about 10-15 minutes.
- Meanwhile, start preparing the avocado pizza sauce. *** (recipe included)
- Once the crust is cooked, add the pizza sauce and any alkaline toppings you wish, such as cherry tomatoes, onions, etc.
- Bake until cooked through, or for a further 15-20 minutes.
- For the pizza sauce
- To make the avocado pizza sauce, first cut the avocado in the middle, discard the stone and then scrape the avocado flesh in a food processor.
- Add all the other sauce ingredients and process until smooth or about 3 minutes.
- Scrape the inside of the food processor once necessary.

71) Alkaline vegan electric chops

Preparation time: **Cooking time:**   **Portions: 1**

Ingredients:
- Grape oil
- 1/2 teaspoon of cayenne
- 1 teaspoon of onion powder
- 1 teaspoon sea salt
- 1/4 cup of spring water
- 2 Portobello mushrooms
- 1/2 cup alkaline barbecue sauce
- For the alkaline electric barbecue sauce
- Servings: approx. 8-10 ounces
- 1/8 teaspoon cloves

Ingredients:
- 1/4 teaspoon cayenne powder
- 1/2 teaspoon ground ginger
- 2 teaspoons of onion powder
- 2 teaspoons of smoked sea salt/sea salt
- 1/4 cup white onions, chopped
- 1/4 cup date sugar
- 2 tablespoons agave
- 6 cherry tomatoes

Directions:
- First, remove the gills from the bottom of the individual mushroom caps and then slice the Portobello about ½ inch apart.
- Place the sauce ingredients in a blender and puree until smooth.
- Add the sliced mushrooms to a container together with the water, a large amount of barbeque sauce and the seasoning.
- Cover the mixture and keep it cool for about 6-8 hours. Be sure to turn it at regular 2-hour intervals.
- Take a skewer and push about 3 Portobello mushrooms around the centre, then take another skewer and repeat. If any slices of mushroom come off, reserve them as ribs.
- Brush a griddle with grapeseed oil and then cook the chops over a medium heat for about 12-15 minutes. Remember to turn them regularly, after every 3 minutes.
- Brush with more sauce after a few throws and serve with your favourite alkaline dish.

72) Walnut meat

Preparation time: **Cooking time:** **Portions: 6**

Ingredients:
- 1/2 cup fresh thyme, chopped
- 1/2 teaspoon of sea salt
- 1 pinch of dried basil

Directions:
- First, soak the nuts in spring water for at least 4 hours, or preferably overnight.
- Add the soaked walnuts to the food processor together with the pepper and onions.
- Add the salt and thyme and process at high speed until the preferred smooth or chunky consistency is achieved.

Ingredients:
- 1 small red onion, chopped
- 1 1/2 cups red pepper, chopped
- 4 cups of soaked walnuts
- Transfer the mixture to a bowl using a rubber spatula and dehydrate to make a nut crumble or meatball.
- You can also add the contents to an airtight container and store it in the fridge for up to 1 week.

73) Electric alkaline steak with mushrooms and cheese

Preparation time: **Cooking time:** **Portions: 4**

Ingredients:

Mushroom mixture:
- 1 teaspoon of savory
- 1 teaspoon of thyme
- 1 teaspoon of oregano
- 1 teaspoon smoked sea salt
- 1 tablespoon onion powder
- 1 tablespoon of grape oil
- 1/2 cup of alkaline electric garlic sauce
- 1 cup of red peppers
- 1 cup green peppers
- 1 cup onions, sliced
- 4 caps of mushrooms

Directions:
- First, slice the mushrooms to about 1/8 inch thickness. Then, in a bowl, whisk the sauce together with the seasonings to make a marinade.
- Immerse the sliced portabella mushrooms in the marinade and leave for about 30 minutes. Stir after about 15 minutes.

Ingredients:

For the cheese:
- 1/2 teaspoon of basil
- 1/2 teaspoon of sea salt
- 1/2 teaspoon of oregano
- 1/2 teaspoon of cayenne powder
- 1 1/2 teaspoons of onion powder
- 1 1/2 teaspoons of hemp seeds
- 1/3 - 1/2 cup of spring water
- 3/4 cup of Brazil nuts, soaked

- To make the 'cheese', mix all the ingredients in a blender until fully incorporated.
- Meanwhile, add the grapeseed oil to a frying pan over medium heat and fry the peppers and onions for about 3-5 minutes.
- Then add the marinated hatches and fry for another 5 minutes. Serve the cheese steak with a bun and enjoy.

74) Alkaline chickpea tofu

Preparation time: **Cooking time:** **Portions: 2**

Ingredients:
- 1 teaspoon of culantro
- 1 teaspoon sea salt

Directions:
- First, line a baking tray with baking paper.
- Then in a saucepan, continuously whisk all of the above ingredients together over medium heat until the oatmeal, or about 3-5 minutes.
- Pour the batter into a baking tray and flatten it with a spatula.

Ingredients:
- 1 cup of chickpea flour
- 2 cups of spring water

- Leave to cool until firm, or for about 30 minutes. You can keep it in the fridge to speed up the process.
- Once it is firm enough, place the tofu on a cutting board and cut it into cubes.
- Serve as is or bake or sauté for a few more minutes. Season as desired and serve.

75) Foo Yung Alkaline Electric Egg

Preparation time: **Cooking time:**   **Portions: 6**

Ingredients:
- Grape oil
- 1 cup of spring water
- 1/8 teaspoon ginger powder
- 1/2 teaspoon of cayenne powder
- 1 teaspoon of oregano
- 1 teaspoon sea salt
- 1 teaspoon of onion powder
- 1 teaspoon of basil

Ingredients:
- 3/4 cup of chickpea flour
- 1/2 cup of red and white onion, chopped
- 1/2 cup green onions, chopped
- 1/2 cup red and green peppers, chopped
- 1 cup butternut squash, chopped
- 2 cups mushrooms, sliced
- 3 cups of prepared spaghetti

Directions:
- Start by whisking the seasonings, chickpea flour and spring water in a bowl.
- Then add the vegetables and the prepared noodles. Mix with your hands until everything is incorporated.
- Using the grapeseed oil, coat a large frying pan well over high heat and then add ½ cup of the pumpkin and vegetable mixture.
- Cut the mixture into patties and cook them in the hot pan until golden brown, or about 3 to 4 minutes on each side. Add more oil if necessary.
- Serve the egg foo yung with fried wild rice and alkaline friendly sauce and enjoy.

76) Alkaline pasta salad

Preparation time: **Cooking time:**   **Portions: 4**

Ingredients:
- 1/4 cup black olives
- 1/2 cup cherry tomatoes, cut in half
- 1/2 cup onions, diced
- 1 cup courgettes/summer courgettes, sliced

Ingredients:
- 1 cup red/yellow/green peppers, diced
- 4 cups of cooked spelt pasta
- 3/4 to 1 cup of alkaline electric 'garlic' sauce

Directions:
- In a large bowl, mix all the ingredients until well incorporated.
- Serve and enjoy.

77) Mushrooms 'Chicken shrimps

Preparation time: **Cooking time:**   **Portions: 6**

Ingredients:
- Grape oil
- 1 teaspoon ground cloves
- 1 teaspoon of cayenne powder
- 2 teaspoons of ginger powder
- 2 teaspoons of onion powder
- 2 teaspoons of sage
- 2 teaspoons of sea salt

Ingredients:
- 2 teaspoons of basil
- 2 teaspoons of oregano
- 1 1/2 cups of spelt flour
- 1 1/2 cups of spring water
- 2-6 portabella, oyster or white mushrooms

Directions:
- First, cut the caps of the portabella, oyster or white mushrooms about 1/2 inch apart and add them to a large bowl. You can also slice the mushroom stems to make nuggets.
- Add some grape seed oil, water and half of the individual seasonings to the bowl and let the mixture marinate for about 1 hour.
- In a separate bowl, mix the rest of the seasonings with the spelt flour and then batter the mushrooms.
- If baking, preheat the oven to 400 degrees F.
- Meanwhile, grease a baking tray with grapeseed oil and then place the mushrooms on the tray.
- Cook each side until crispy, turning once, or about 15 minutes per side. Serve.
- If using a cooker, heat a frying pan over medium-high heat. Then add about 3 tablespoons of grapeseed oil to the pan.
- Cook the mushrooms until they are crispy, or for about 3 to 4 minutes per side. Be careful not to let the oil burst due to the high heat or liquid from the mushrooms. Enjoy your meal!

78) Pizza Margarita

Preparation time: **Cooking time:** **Portions: 6**

Ingredients:
Crust:
- 1 1/2 cups of spelt flour
- 1 cup of spring water
- 1/2 teaspoon onion powder
- 1/2 teaspoon of oregano
- 1/2 teaspoon of sea salt
- 1/2 teaspoon of basil

Cheese:
- 1/4 teaspoon sea salt
- 1/2 teaspoon of basil
- 1/2 teaspoon of oregano

Directions:
- In a medium bowl, combine all the seasonings with the spelt flour and then add half a cup of water.
- Add more water in small amounts until the dough becomes a ball, or add more spelt flour if you find the dough moist.
- Roll the dough on a floured surface, in one direction as you turn it, and turn it over after a couple of rolls. Keep adding spelt flour after turning to prevent the dough from becoming too sticky.
- Place the dough in a pan lightly coated with oil, making holes with a fork, and now bake in a preheated oven at 350 degrees for about 10-15 minutes.

Ingredients:
- 1/2 teaspoon onion powder
- 1 teaspoon lime juice
- 1/4 cup hemp/walnut milk
- 1/2 cup of spring water
- 1 cup of Brazil nuts, soaked for more than 2 hours

Seals:
- Alkaline electric tomato sauce
- Red onion, sliced
- Plum tomatoes, sliced

- Meanwhile, add all the ingredients for the cheese to a blender and process until smooth, or about 1 or 2 minutes.
- As soon as the crust is cooked, put the cheese, alkaline sauce and your favourite toppings on top. Add more cheese and sauce if you like.
- Cook the contents on the bottom of the grill at 425 degrees F for another 10-15 minutes. Enjoy your meal!!!

79) Vegetarian electric alkaline lasagne

Preparation time: **Cooking time:**   **Portions: 6**

Ingredients:
Pasta
- ✓ Spelt lasagne sheets
- ✓ Tomato sauce
- ✓ 1/2 teaspoon of cayenne powder
- ✓ 2 teaspoons of sea salt
- ✓ 2 teaspoons of oregano
- ✓ 2 teaspoons of basil
- ✓ 1 tablespoon onion powder
- ✓ 1 tablespoon agave
- ✓ 12 plumcake tomatoes
- ✓ "Meat alternative
- ✓ 1 teaspoon fennel powder
- ✓ 2 teaspoons of basil
- ✓ 2 teaspoons of oregano
- ✓ 1 tablespoon sea salt
- ✓ 2 tablespoons of onion powder

Ingredients:
- ✓ 1/2 cup of tomato sauce
- ✓ 1 cup diced green, yellow and red peppers
- ✓ 1 cup onions, chopped
- ✓ 1 cup of cooked chickpeas (garbanzo beans)
- ✓ 2 cups of cooked spelt berries/kernels
- ✓ Brazil nut cheese
- ✓ 1 teaspoon of basil
- ✓ 1 teaspoon of oregano
- ✓ 1 teaspoon sea salt
- ✓ 1 tablespoon onion powder
- ✓ 1 tablespoon hemp seeds
- ✓ 1 cup of spring water
- ✓ 2 cups of soaked Brazil nuts
- ✓ Extra
- ✓ White mushrooms
- ✓ Grape oil
- ✓ Courgettes

Directions:
- ❖ Add the ingredients for the tomato sauce to a blender and then process until well combined.
- ❖ Add the grapeseed oil to a saucepan with the tomato sauce and heat the sauce over a medium heat. Lower the heat and simmer until the sauce has thickened, or for 2 hours, stirring regularly.
- ❖ In a food processor, combine the ingredients for the 'meat' which are the chickpea beans, spelt and seasonings until well incorporated.
- ❖ Lightly coat a frying pan with oil and heat it over a medium heat. Fry the peppers and onions for about 5 minutes.
- ❖ Now add the chickpea and spelt mixture from the food processor and a little grapeseed oil to the pan and cook the mixture until it starts to brown, or for 10-12 minutes.
- ❖ In a blender, add the remaining cheese ingredients along with 1 cup of water and process until well combined. If you find it too thick, add ¼ cup of spring water at a time until you get the desired consistency.
- ❖ Reserve one cup of tomato sauce, and then pour the rest of the sauce into the chickpea and spelt mixture. Combine well.
- ❖ Slice the courgettes and mushrooms lengthwise. You can also make lasagne with courgettes instead of spelt pasta, if you like.
- ❖ At this point, start preparing the lasagne. Lightly coat the bottom of the dish with the reserved tomato sauce to ensure that it does not stick.
- ❖ Then the spelt paste, sliced courgettes, chickpea and spelt mixture, alkaline cheese, white mushrooms and spelt paste are spread out.
- ❖ Repeat this arrangement until you have 4 layers of dough. Then, cover the last layer with the chickpea and spelt mixture and the cheese.
- ❖ Pour the rest of the tomato sauce around the layers of lasagne and sprinkle with a little dried basil if you like.
- ❖ Bake at 350 degrees F for about 35-45 minutes.
- ❖ Then leave the lasagne to cool for about 15 minutes and serve.

80) **Stuffed aubergines**

Preparation time: **Cooking time:**   **Portions: 6**

Ingredients:
- Cayenne pepper
- Sea salt
- 2 tablespoons of tomato puree
- 1 teaspoon ground cumin
- 1 teaspoon agave
- 1 cup chopped cherry tomatoes
- 1 green pepper, seeded and chopped

Directions:
- Preheat the oven to 450 degrees F and then place a rack in the centre of the oven.
- Line a baking tray with baking paper or aluminium foil and brush with a little olive oil.
- Then remove the wide strips of aubergine skin using a peeler. Cut the aubergine lengthways, but do not slice it completely.
- Now sprinkle a pinch of salt into each and then place in a colander for about 30 minutes.
- Place them on the baking tray and bake until the outer skins begin to roar, about 20 minutes. Remove from the oven and cool.
- Meanwhile, heat 2 tablespoons of olive oil in a large frying pan over medium heat and add the onions.

Ingredients:
- 2 medium-sized red onions, chopped
- 3 tablespoons chopped fresh sage/basil
- 1 fennel bulb, chopped
- 4 tablespoons of olive oil, divided by
- 6 thin aubergines

- Cook for a few minutes, stirring occasionally, and then add the fennel and pepper. Cook for about 10 minutes, or until the vegetables are tender and have collapsed.
- Season the mixture with salt and cayenne pepper then mix with parsley, tomato puree, cumin, sugar and chopped tomato.
- Cook until fragrant, about 5 minutes. Set aside. Lower oven temperature to 350 degrees F.
- In a baking dish, arrange the aubergines so that each one is open with butter. Season with salt and fill with the tomato and onion mixture.
- Drizzle with the rest of the olive oil, and then add two tablespoons of water to the pan. Cook until the aubergines are flat and the liquid in the pan has caramelised, about 40-45 minutes.
- Serve the aubergines hot or at room temperature, preferably with the cooking juices poured over the aubergines.

81) **Quinoa pasta with tomato sauce and artichokes**

Preparation time: **Cooking time:**   **Portions: 2**

Ingredients:
- 2 tablespoons cold-pressed extra virgin olive oil
- 1 pinch of cayenne pepper
- 1/2 teaspoon sea salt, organic
- 3 tablespoons of fresh basil
- 1 teaspoon unleavened vegetable stock
- 1 ounce of walnuts

Directions:
- Cook the artichoke until tender.
- Then cook the pasta according to the package instructions. While it is cooking, dice the tomatoes, and then chop up the basil, fennel and onion.
- In a frying pan, heat 2 tablespoons of olive oil and fry the onions, walnuts and fennel for a few minutes.

Ingredients:
- 1 fennel bulb
- 1 medium-sized onion
- 8 ounces of artichoke hearts, fresh or frozen
- 5 ounces of cherry tomatoes, fresh
- 7 ounces of quinoa or spelt pasta

- Then add the cooked artichoke hearts and tomatoes and cook for 2 minutes.
- Collect about 1/2 cup of water and then dissolve the vegetable stock in the water. Add to a pan. Simmer for 2 minutes over a low heat, stirring regularly.
- Finally, add the basil and season with salt and cayenne pepper. To serve, pour the sauce over the pasta.

82) Sautéed mushrooms

Preparation time: **Cooking time:** **Portions: 6**

Ingredients:
- ✓ 1 fennel bulb, chopped
- ✓ ½ lemons
- ✓ 1 ½ teaspoons of sea salt
- ✓ 3 tablespoons of extra virgin olive oil

Ingredients:
- ✓ 2 tablespoons sage, chopped
- ✓ 1/4 teaspoon cayenne pepper
- ✓ 24 ounces of fresh mushrooms

Directions:
- ❖ Immerse the mushrooms in water and shake them to clean them well, and drain them completely. Cut and slice the mushrooms into bite-sized pieces.
- ❖ Place the mushrooms in a bowl and squeeze in the juice of the half a lemon. Stir to combine.
- ❖ In a large frying pan, add the fennel and then pour in the olive oil.
- ❖ Heat the mixture over medium-high heat until the fennel starts to sizzle; this should take about 30 seconds.
- ❖ Now add the mushrooms, stir and cover. Continue cooking, stirring occasionally; say at intervals of about 4 minutes.
- ❖ Once cooked, remove the lid and add a little salt and cayenne pepper and continue cooking. After about 5 minutes, the mushrooms should start to brown and all the moisture should have evaporated.
- ❖ Now stir in the sage and then serve the delicious meal. Enjoy your meal!

83) Electric alkaline flat bread

Preparation time: **Cooking time:** **Portions: 4**

Ingredients:
- ✓ 1/4 teaspoon of cayenne
- ✓ 2 teaspoons of onion powder
- ✓ 2 teaspoons of basil
- ✓ 2 teaspoons of oregano

Ingredients:
- ✓ 1 tablespoon sea salt
- ✓ 3/4 cup of spring water
- ✓ 2 tablespoons of grape oil
- ✓ 2 cups of spelt flour

Directions:
- ❖ Start by combining all the seasonings and flour together until well incorporated.
- ❖ Then add ½ cup of water and the oil and mix well until the mixture becomes a ball.
- ❖ Put some flour on the work area and now knead the dough for about 5 minutes. Divide the dough into 6 portions.
- ❖ Roll the individual balls into circles of about 4 inches. Place the balls in a frying pan and cook over a medium heat until cooked through, turning after about 3 minutes.
- ❖ Serve with curry.

84) Alkaline dinner plate

Preparation time: **Cooking time:** **Portions: 4**

Ingredients:
- ✓ Cabbage dish
- ✓ 1/2 cup chopped red onions
- ✓ 1/4 habanero pepper
- ✓ 2 tablespoons agave
- ✓ Sea salt
- ✓ 1/2 cup green onions
- ✓ 1 cup of chopped orange, yellow and sweet red peppers
- ✓ 2 bunches of green cabbage
- ✓ Pasta dish
- ✓ 1/2 teaspoon of grape oil
- ✓ 1/2 cup chopped yellow pumpkin
- ✓ 1/4 cup chopped red and green peppers

Ingredients:
- ✓ 1 teaspoon sea salt
- ✓ 1/4 cup chopped green and red onions
- ✓ 1 cup chopped portabella mushrooms
- ✓ 1 tin of Kamut pasta
- ✓ Fried oyster mushrooms
- ✓ Sea salt to taste
- ✓ ½ cup of spelt flour
- ✓ A pinch of cayenne pepper
- ✓ ½ teaspoon of onion powder
- ✓ 1/2 king oyster mushroom, large
- ✓ Avocado slices, optional

Directions:
- ❖ Clean the cabbage and cut it into small pieces. Gently coat the bottom of a pan with grapeseed oil and add the peppers and onions.
- ❖ Fry the vegetables for a few seconds then add the cabbage and agave. Cook the mixture over a medium heat, stirring regularly, for about 30 minutes.
- ❖ Now bring the water to the boil in a saucepan and add ½ teaspoon of oil and a teaspoon of salt. Add the kamut pasta
- ❖ Fry peppers, onions and portabella mushrooms in a frying pan for a few minutes.
- ❖ Add the cooked kamut paste to the vegetables together with the shredded pumpkin. Stir well.
- ❖ Now rinse the oyster mushrooms, season with cayenne pepper, onion powder and sea salt.
- ❖ Coat the mushrooms with spelt flour and fry in oil. Once cooked, remove from heat and place on a towel to absorb the extra oil.
- ❖ Serve while still warm.

85) Bowl of alkaline Tahini noodles

Preparation time: **Cooking time:** **Portions: 2**

Ingredients:
- Bowl
- 1 teaspoon black sesame seeds
- 1/2 avocado, sliced
- 2 green onions, chopped
- 4 cabbages, chopped
- 1 parsnip, chopped
- 4 turbot leaves, chopped

Directions:
- Slice, chop and mince the vegetables as indicated above, add to a bowl.
- Add all the ingredients for the dressing to another small bowl and whisk until fully combined.

Ingredients:
- 1 yellow courgette, spiralised
- Condiment
- 1 teaspoon of agave or any other liquid sweetener
- 2 tablespoons of lemon juice
- 1 tablespoon tahini
- A pinch of salt

- Pour the dressing over the vegetables and garnish with sesame seeds.

86) Balancing alkaline salad

Preparation time: **Cooking time:** **Portions: 4**

Ingredients:
- 1 tablespoon sesame seeds
- 1 tablespoon diced spring onion
- 1/4 cup of chopped culantro
- 1/2 cup of chopped alfalfa sprouts
- 1/2 cup of chopped snow pea shoots
- 1/2 avocado
- 5 red radishes
- 1 cup chopped rocket

Directions:
- Mix all the ingredients for the dressing in a large bowl until combined.
- Wash and trim the edges of the green beans.
- Add the green beans to a saucepan and add enough water to cover them almost completely. Cook over a low heat until they are almost tender, or for about 3 minutes.
- Remove the green beans from the heat and leave them to drain. Then cut the green beans into 1-inch pieces.

Ingredients:
- 10 green beans
- Condiment
- 1 teaspoon green mustard
- 1 tablespoon olive oil
- 1 tablespoon lemon juice
- 1/4 teaspoon Celtic sea salt
- Cayenne pepper, to taste

- Now slice the radishes and finely chop the spring onion, culantro and snow pea shoots.
- Pull the alfafa sprouts by hand and then put all the chopped ingredients in a large bowl together with the seasoning.
- Serve the salad topped with half of the avocado. Alternatively, you can also chop the avocado and fold it slowly into the salad.
- Sprinkle with a few sesame seeds and serve the salad garnished with lemon juice.

SNACKs

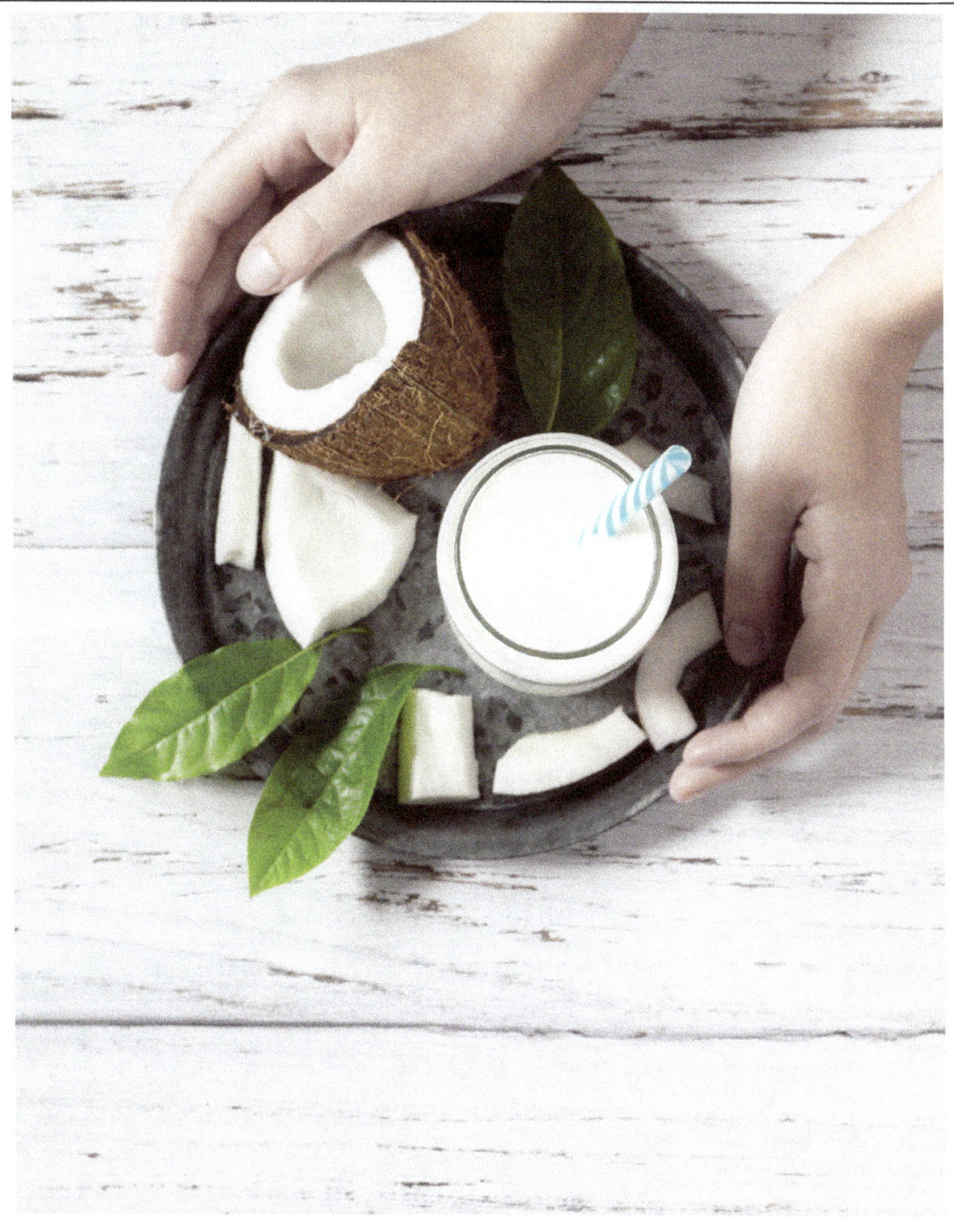

87) Spicy Toasted nuts

Preparation time: 10 minutes. **Cooking time:** 15 minutes. **Portions: 4**

Ingredients:
- 8 ounces of pecans or coconuts or walnuts
- 1 teaspoon sea salt
- 1 tablespoon olive oil or coconut oil

Directions:
- Add all the ingredients to an oven. Fry the nuts until golden brown.

Ingredients:
- 1 teaspoon of ground cumin
- 1 teaspoon paprika powder or chili powder

- Serve and enjoy.

88) Wheat Crackers

Preparation time: 10 minutes. **Cooking time:** 20 minutes. **Portions: 4**

Ingredients:
- 1 3/4 cups of walnut flour
- 1 1/2 cups coconut flour
- 3/4 teaspoon sea salt

Directions:
- Set your oven to 350 degrees F.
- Mix the coconut flour, walnut flour and salt in a bowl.
- Stir in vegetable oil and salt. Stir well until cooked.
- Pour the dough onto a flat surface in a thin dish.

Ingredients:
- 1/3 vegetable oil
- 1 kitchen basket
- Sea salt for sprinkling
- Cut small squares out of the sheet.
- Place the squares of dough on a sheet of baking paper lined with parchment paper.
- Wet for 20 minutes until the light comes on.
- Serve.

89) Chips potato

Preparation time: 10 mnutes. **Cooking time:** 5 minutes. **Portions: 4**

Ingredients:
- 1 tablespoon vegetable oil

Directions:
- Toss potato with oil and sea salt.
- Distribute the slices in a sandwich dish in a single row.

Ingredients:
- 1 potato, sliced paper thin Sea salt, to taste
- Bake for 5 minutes until golden brown.
- Serve.

90) Courgette Pepper Chips

Preparation time: 10 minutes. **Cooking time:** 15 minutes. **Portions: 4**

Ingredients:
- 1 2/3 cups vegetable oil
- 1 teaspoon onion powder
- 1/2 teaspoon of black pepper

Directions:
- Mix the oil with all the spices in a bowl.
- Add the zucchini slices and mix well.
- Transfer the mixture in a Zip lock container and seal il.

Ingredients:
- 3 tablespoons crushed red pepper flakes
- 2 courgette, thinly sliced

- Refrigerate for 10 minutes.
- Spread the zucchini slices on a greased baking tray.
- Bake for 15 minutes
- Serve.

91) Flat bread

Preparation time: **Cooking time:** 20 Minutes   **Portions: 6**

Ingredients:
- 2 cups of Spelt Flour
- 2 teaspoons of Oregano
- 2 teaspoons of Onion powder
- 1/4 teaspoon of Cayenne

Ingredients:
- 2 teaspoons of basil
- 1 tablespoon of Pure Sea Salt
- 3/4 cup o of spring water
- 2 tablespoons of Grape seed oil

Directions:
- Add the spelt flour and all the cereals to a bowl and mix well.
- Add the Grape Seed Oil and 1/2 cup of Spring Water and continue to mix.
- Try to form a thick ball. If it is too thick, add more Spring Water.
- Make a place to roll the mud and sprinkle it with flour.
- Knead the dough for about 5 minutes until it has become desired consistencyn.
- Divide the dough in 6 equal balls.
- Roll out each loaf in a circles container about 4 inches in diameter.
- Prepare a wooden frying pan. Put one flatbred in the pan and cook over a medium heat.
- Turn the dish upside down for 2 to 3 minutes and work until dry. Small pieces of sugar paper should be placed on both sides.
- Keep looking at the upper body.
- Serve and enjoy your Flatbread!

Helpful hints: You can add seasonings according to your taste.

92) Cracker Healthy

Preparation time: **Cooking time:** 30 minutes   **Portions: 50 Crackers**

Ingredients:
- 1/2 cup of rye flour
- 1 cup Spelt flour
- 2 teaspoons of Sesame Seed
- 1 teaspoon of Agave Syrup

Ingredients:
- 1 teaspoon of Pure Sea Salt
- 2 tablespoons of Grape Seed Oil
- 3/4 cup of Spring Water

Directions:
- Preheat our oven to 350 degrees Fahrenheit.
- Add all the ingredients to a glass container and mix everything together.
- Make a ball of dough. If the dough is too thick, add more flour.
- Prepare a place to spread the dough and cover it with a piece of parchment paper.
- Degrease the container well with Grape Seed Oil and place the dart in it.
- RETARD the slurry with a rolling pin, adding more flour to keep it from falling apart.
- When your dough is ready, take a pastry cutter and insert it into the container. If you don't have a pastry cutter, you can use a biscuit cutter.
- Arrange the squares on a kitchen basket and place them in the corner of a ech square using a fork of a skewer.
- Brush the plate with a little cereal oil and sprinkle with a little pure sea salt if necessary.
- Bake for 12-15 minutes or until the crackers are golden brown.
- Everything that was done was done with the help of another person.
- Serve and enjoy your Healthy Crackers!

Helpful hints: You can add any seasonings from the Doctor Sebi's food list as per your wish. You can make the crackers with our tomato sauce, avocado sauce or cheese. Sauce.

93) Tortillas

Preparation time:.   **Cooking time:** 20 Minutes   **Portions: 8**

Ingredients:
- 2 cups Spelt flour
- 1 teaspoon of Pure Sea Salt

Ingredients:
- 1/2 cup of spring Water

Directions:
- In a food processor* mix the spelt flour with pure salt. Blend for about 15 minutes.
- Blend, slowly add the Grape seed oil until well distributed.
- Slowly add the soy water, stirring until a colour forms.
- Prepare a piece of wallpaper and pour some parchment paper over it. Sprinkle with a little flour.
- Process the stock cube for about 1 to 2 minutes until it reaches the right consistency.
- Pour the dough into 8-inch pieces.
- Roll the sandwich into a very thin shape.
- Prepare a lunchbox, cook one tortilla at a time in the microwave for about 30-60 minutes.
- Serve and enjoy your Tortillas!

Useful tips: If you do not have a refrigerator, you can use a mixer or blender. However, you'll get a better result with a food as you have nothing to do with. You can serve the Tortillas with our Sweet Butter Sauce, Avocado Sauce or Cheese. Sauce.

94) Tortilla chips

Preparation time: **Cooking time:** 30 minutes **Portions:** 8

Ingredients:
- ✓ 2 cups of Spelt Flour
- ✓ 1 teaspoon of Pure Sea Salt

Directions:
- ❖ Set the oven to 350 degrees Fahrenheit.
- ❖ Place the spelt flour and pure salt in a food processor*. Blend for about 15 seconds.
- ❖ While stirring, slowly add the soya oil until well combined.
- ❖ Continue to blend and slowly add Spring Water to a dough is formed.
- ❖ Prepare a work surface and cover it with a piece of parchment paper. Sprinkle flour over it.
- ❖ Knead the dough for about 1 to 2 minutes, until it is just right.
- ❖ Cover a baking pan with a little Grape Sed Oil.

Ingredients:
- ✓ 1/2 cup of rinse water
- ✓ 1/3 cup of ground olive oil
- ❖ Place the prepared dart in the baking tray.
- ❖ Brush the mixture with a little grape oil and, if desired, a little pure sea salt.
- ❖ Cut the dough into 8 pieces with a pizza knife.
- ❖ Bake for about 10-12 minutes or until the chips are starting toecome golden brown.
- ❖ Allow to cool before serving.
- ❖ Serve and enjoy your Tortilla Chips!

Useful tips: If you do not have a refrigerator, you can use a hand mixer or a blender. However, you will get better results with an immersion blender. You can serve the Tortillas with our Sweet Barbecue Sauce, Guacamole, or "Cheese". Sauce .

95) Onion Rings

Preparation time: **Cooking time:** 30 Minutes. **Portions:** 8

Ingredients:
- ✓ White or yellow onion
- ✓ 1 cup of Spelt Flour
- ✓ 1/2 cup of homemade Hempseed Milk
- ✓ 1/2 cup of Aquafaba *
- ✓ 2 teaspoons of Onion Powder.

Directions:
- ❖ Preheat our oven to 450 degrees Fahrenheit.
- ❖ Pour Homemade Hempseed Milk and Aquafaba into a medium bowl and mix well.
- ❖ Add 1 teaspoon of Oregano, 1 teaspoon of Onion Powder, 1/2 teaspoon of Cayenne, and 1 teaspoon of Pure Sea Salt to the wet ingredients and mix.
- ❖ Peel the Onions, slice the ends.
- ❖ Cut the peeled onion into slices about 1/4 inch thick. Cut the onion into rings.
- ❖ Add the Spelt flour, 1 teaspoon of Oregano, 1 teaspoon of Onion Powder, 1/2 teact of Cayenne, and 1
- ❖ taspoon of Pure Sea Salt in a container with a quart. Shake out all the liquid.

Ingredients:
- ✓ 2 teaspoons of Oregano
- ✓ 1 teaspoon of Cayenne powder
- ✓ 2 teaspoons of Pure Sea Salt
- ✓ 3 tablespoons of grape oil

- ❖ Brush a baking sheet with Grape Seed Oil 8. Place a couple onion rings over the water mixture.
- ❖ Put the water onion rings in the dry mixture and turn till coated on both sides.
- ❖ Place the covered onion rings on the baking tray.
- ❖ Repeat steps from 8 to 10 until all onion rings are covere.
- ❖ Lightly spray the rings with Grape seed oil.
- ❖ Water for about 10-15 minutes until it glows.
- ❖ This is possible for coool them before serving.
- ❖ Serve and enjoy our onion rings!

Helpful Hints: If you haven't made Aquafaba, add 1/2 extra millet of Homemade hemp seed milk. You can use Onion Rings with our sweet Bärbecue Sauce , or "Cheese" Sauce .

DESSERTS

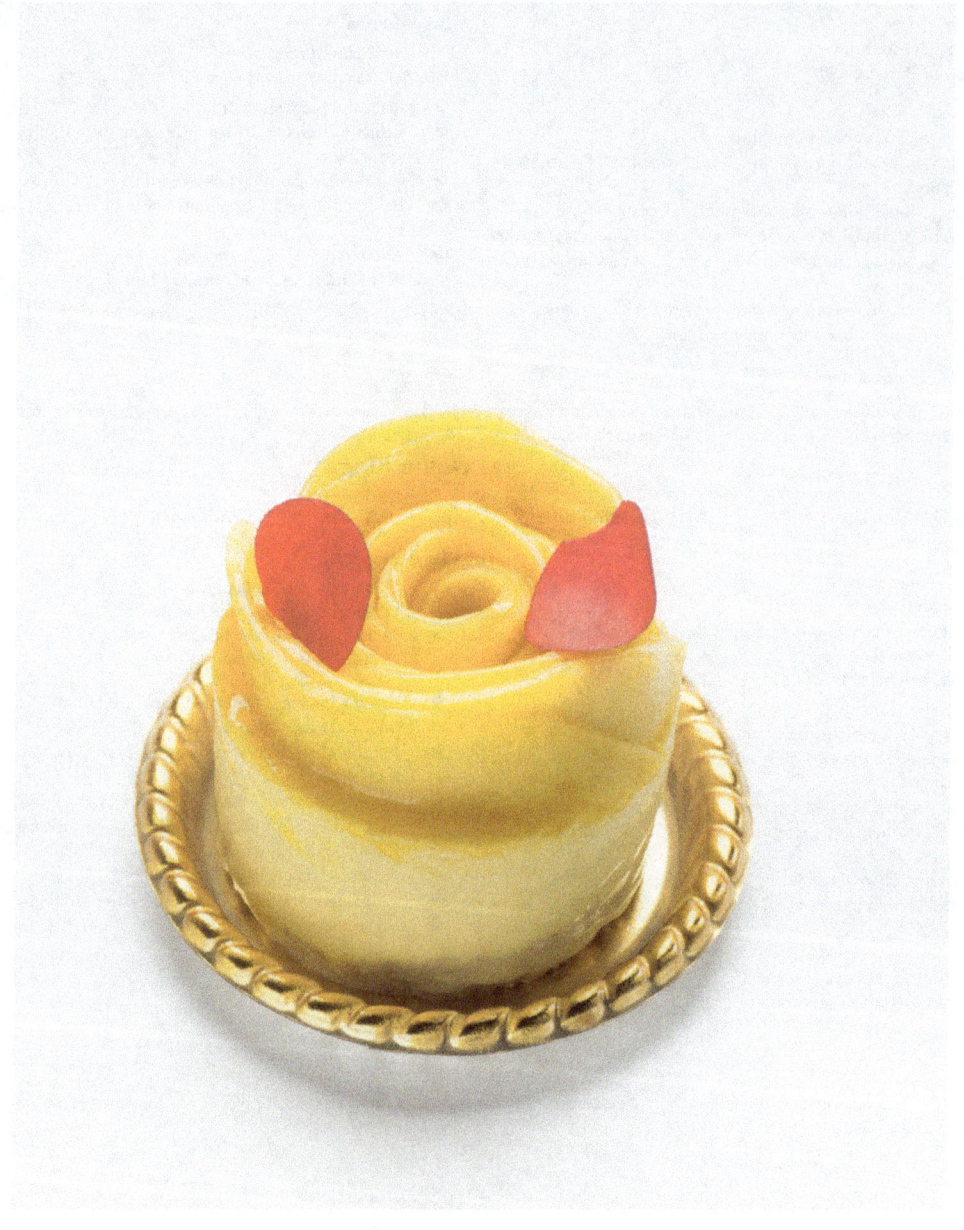

96) Green apple smoothie

Preparation time: 10 minutes

Cooking time: 0 minutes

Portions: 1

Ingredients:
- ✓ 1 peach, peeled and pitted
- ✓ 1 green apple, peeled and cored

Directions:
- ❖ Add all ingredients to a blender.

Ingredients:
- ✓ 1 cup of alkaline water

- ❖ Blend well until smooth.
- ❖ Serve with apple slices.

97) Avocado smoothie

Preparation time: 10 minutes

Cooking time: 0 minutes

Portions: 1

Ingredients:
- ✓ 1 carrot, grated
- ✓ 1 avocado, with stone and skin
- ✓ ½ pear, core

Directions:
- ❖ Add all ingredients to a blender.
- ❖ Blend well until smooth.

Ingredients:
- ✓ ½ cup blackberries
- ✓ 1 ½ cups unsweetened almond milk

- ❖ Serve with blackberries on top.

98) Green smoothie

Preparation time: 10 minutes

Cooking time: 0 minutes

Portions: 1

Ingredients:
- ✓ 1 cup of alkaline water
- ✓ 3/4 cup raw coconut water
- ✓ 1/2 teaspoon of probiotic powder
- ✓ 2 cups of well-packed spinach
- ✓ 1 cup of raw young Thai coconut meat
- ✓ 1 avocado, peeled and stoned
- ✓ 1/2 cucumber, cut into small pieces

Directions:
- ❖ Add all ingredients to a blender.

Ingredients:
- ✓ 1 teaspoon of lime zest, finely grated
- ✓ 2 limes, hav
- ✓ led
- ✓ Stevia, as desired
- ✓ Pinch of Celtic sea salt
- ✓ 2 cups of ice cubes

- ❖ Blend well until smooth.
- ❖ Serve with a slice of avocado on top.

99) Oatmeal and orange smoothie

Preparation time: 10 minutes **Cooking time**: **Portions**: 4

Ingredients:
- 2/3 cups rolled oats
- 2 oranges, peeled, seeded and cut into sections
- 2 large bananas, peeled and sliced

Directions:
- Place all ingredients in a high-speed blender and pulse until creamy.

Ingredients:
- 2 cups unsweetened almond milk
- 1 cup ice cubes, crushed

- Pour the smoothie into four glasses and serve immediately.

100) Spicy banana smoothie

Preparation time: 5 minutes **Cooking time**: 5 minutes **Portions**: 2

Ingredients:
- 2 medium-sized frozen bananas, peeled and sliced
- 1 teaspoon organic vanilla extract
- ¼ teaspoon ground cinnamon

Directions:
- Place all ingredients in a high-speed blender and pulse until creamy.

Ingredients:
- Pinch of ground nutmeg
- Pinch of ground cloves
- 1½ cups unsweetened almond milk

- Pour the smoothie into two glasses and serve immediately.

101) Blueberry smoothie

Preparation time: 5 minutes **Cooking time**: 5 minutes **Portions**: 2

Ingredients:
- 2 cups of frozen blueberries
- 1½ cups unsweetened almond milk

Directions:
- Place all ingredients in a high-speed blender and pulse until creamy.

Ingredients:
- 1 small banana, peeled and sliced
- ¼ cup ice cubes

- Serve immediately after pouring the smoothie into two glasses.

102) Raspberry and tofu smoothie

Preparation time: 10 minutes **Cooking time**: **Portions**: 2

Ingredients:
- 8 ounces of firm, pressed and drained silken tofu
- 1 cup frozen raspberries
- ¼ tablespoon of coconut extract

Directions:
- Place all ingredients in a high-speed blender and pulse until creamy.

Ingredients:
- 4-6 drops of liquid stevia
- 1 cup of coconut cream
- ½ cup ice cubes, crushed

- Pour the smoothie into two glasses and serve immediately.

103) Papaya smoothie

Preparation time: 10 minutes **Cooking time:** **Portions:** 2

Ingredients:
- 1 large banana, peeled and sliced
- ½ medium papaya, peeled and roughly chopped
- 1½ cups unsweetened almond milk
- 2 tablespoons agave syrup

Directions:
- Place all ingredients in a high-speed blender and pulse until creamy.

Ingredients:
- 1 tablespoon fresh lime juice
- ¼ teaspoon ground turmeric
- ½ cup ice cubes, crushed

- Pour the smoothie into two glasses and serve immediately.

104) Peach smoothie

Preparation time: **Cooking time:** **Portions:** 2

Ingredients:
- 1 large peach, peeled, pitted and chopped
- 1 medium frozen banana, peeled and sliced
- 2 ounces of aloe vera
- ½ teaspoon of fresh ginger, peeled and chopped

Directions:
- Add all ingredients to a high-speed blender and pulse until smooth.

Ingredients:
- 2 tablespoons of linseed
- ½ teaspoon organic vanilla extract
- 1¾ cup unsweetened almond milk

- Pour the smoothie into two glasses and serve immediately.

105) Strawberry and beetroot smoothie

Preparation time: 10 minutes **Cooking time:** **Portions:** 2

Ingredients:
- 2 cups of frozen strawberries, stoned and chopped
- 2/3 cup frozen beetroot, chopped
- 1 teaspoon fresh ginger, peeled and grated

Directions:
- Add all ingredients to a high-speed blender and pulse until smooth.

Ingredients:
- 1 teaspoon fresh turmeric, peeled and grated
- ½ cup of fresh orange juice
- 1 cup unsweetened almond milk

- Pour the smoothie into two glasses and serve immediately.

106) Grape and chard smoothie

Preparation time: 10 minutes **Cooking time:** **Portions:** 2

Ingredients:
- 2 cups of seedless green grapes
- 2 cups fresh beetroot, cut and chopped
- 2 tablespoons agave nectar

Directions:
- Add all ingredients to a high-speed blender and pulse until smooth.

Ingredients:
- 1 teaspoon fresh lemon juice
- 1½ cups of alkaline water
- ¼ cup ice cubes, crushed

- Pour the smoothie into two glasses and serve immediately.

AUTHOR BIBLIOGRAPHY

THE ESSENCIAL ALKALINE DIET COOKBOOK FOR BEGINNERS

100+ Alkaline Recipes to Bring Your Body Back to Balance! Healthy Recipes to Enjoy Favorite Foods for Weight-Loss!

THE ALKAINE HEALTHY DIET FOR WOMEN

The Effective Way to Follow an Alkaline Diet comprising Plant-Based Diet Recipes: Natural Ways To Prevent Diabetes! 100+ Recipes Included!

THE ALKAINE HEALTHY DIET FOR MEN

100+ Recipes to Understand pH, Eat Well, and Reclaim Your Health! Plant-Based Recipes Are Included! Boost your Weight-Loss!

THE ALKAINE HEALTHY DIET FOR KIDS

100+ Recipes for Your Health, To Lose Weight Naturally and Bring Your Body Back To Balance

THE ALKALINE FIET COOKBOOK FOR ONE

100+ Recipes to Lose Weight and Get the Benefits of an Alkaline Diet - Alkaline Smoothies Included for Your Way to Vibrant Health - Massive Energy and Natural Weight Loss! Plant-Based Recipes Are Included!

THE ALKAINE DIET FOR WOMEN AFTER 50

2 Books in 1: The Complete Alkaline Diet Guidebook for Beginners: Understand pH, Eat Well with Easy Alkaline Diet Cookbook and more than 200+ Delicious Recipes (Lose weight, Beginners, Foods & Diet, Reset Cleanse)

THE SPECIAL ALKALINE DIET FOR TWO

2 Books in 1: Guidebook for Beginners: Understand pH, Eat Well with Easy Alkaline Diet Cookbook and more than 200 Delicious Recipes! Plant-Based Recipes Are Included!

THE ALKALINE DIET FOR DADDY AND SON

2 Books in 1: For Beginners: The Ultimate Guide of Alkaline Herbal Medicine for permanent weight loss, Understand pH with 200+ Anti Inflammatory Recipes Cookbook! Plant-Based Recipes Are Included!

THE ALKALINE DIET FAST & EASY

2 Books in 1: The Complete and Exhaustive Beginner's Guide to lose Weight, Fasting and Revitalize Your Body with Plant-Based Diet including 200+ Healthy and Tasty Recipes!

THE ALKALINE DIET FOR MUM AND KIDDOS

2 Books in 1: The Simplest Alkaline Diet Guide for Beginners + 200 Easy Recipes: How to Cure Your Body, Lose Weight and Regain Your Life with Easy Alkaline Diet Cookbook! Plant-Based Recipes Are Included!

THE ALKALINE DIET TO LOSE WEIGHT FAST

3 Books in 1: The Revolution of Eating Habits to stay Healthy and Find the Best Shape. A complete Program with 300+ Recipes to Regain a Healthy Balance of the Body with Alkaline Foods and lose Weight Quickly.

THE ALKALINE DIET FOR A HEALTHY FAMILY

3 Books in 1: A Complete Guide for Beginners to Clean and Treat Your Body, Eat Well with More Than 300+ Easy Alkaline Recipes for Weight Loss and Fight Chronic Disease!

THE ALKALINE DIET HIGH-PROTEIN FOR SPORT PLAYERS

3 Books in 1: Diet for Beginners: Top 300+ Alkaline Recipes for Weight Loss with Plant Based Diet And 21 Secrets To Reset And Understand pH Right Now!

THE ALKALINE DIET FOR ABSOLUTE BEGINNERS

3 Books in 1: This Cookbook Includes: Alkaline Diet for Beginners + Alkaline Diet Cookbook, The Best Guidebook to Understanding pH Secrets with More Than 300+ Recipes for Weight Loss and Anti-Inflammatory Action!

THE ALKALINE DIET COMPLETE EDITION FOR EVERYBODY

4 Books in 1: The complete guide to eat well and Lose Weight while understanding pH and prevent disease to boost your everyday energy! 400+ Recipes with Plant-Based Recipes Included!

CONCLUSIONS

Congratulations! You made it to the end!

Thank you for making it to the end of the Alkaline Diet; we hope it was informative and provided all you need to reach your goals, whatever they may be.

With the information you have, you can now start a successful alkaline diet. Your body works best when it's not acidic. The alkaline diet ensures that your body functions at its best. The great thing is that all the food you can eat is tasty. With the recipes in this book, you won't have to worry about making dinner. So don't wait any longer. Start today, and you will see your body change for the better.

The purpose of this cookbook was to introduce readers to most of the insights regarding the alkaline diet in a comprehensive way. Therefore, the text of this book has been categorized into several sections, each of which discusses the basics, the details, what it has and what it doesn't, and recipes related to the alkaline diet. In addition, the recipe chapter is divided into subsections, ranging from breakfast to lunch, dinner, smoothies, snacks, and desserts. So take some time to travel the length of this book and experience the miraculous effects of an alkaline diet on your mind and health.

Laura Green

Laura Green

www.ingramcontent.com/pod-product-compliance
Lightning Source LLC
Chambersburg PA
CBHW081422080526
44589CB00016B/2632